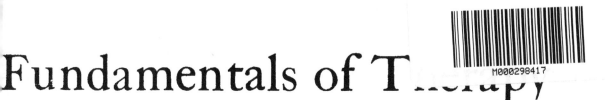

Fundamentals of Therapy

An Extension of the Art of Healing
through Spiritual Knowledge

By

Rudolf Steiner, Ph.D.

and

Ita Wegman, M.D. (Zurich)

Authorized Translation from
the German

London
Anthroposophical Publishing Co.
46 Gloucester Place, W.1

1925

Kessinger Publishing's Rare Reprints
Thousands of Scarce and Hard-to-Find Books!

·   ·   ·
·   ·   ·
·   ·   ·
·   ·   ·
·   ·   ·
·   ·   ·
·   ·   ·
·   ·   ·
·   ·   ·
·   ·   ·
·   ·   ·
·   ·   ·
·   ·   ·
·   ·   ·
·   ·   ·
·   ·   ·
·   ·   ·
·   ·   ·
·   ·   ·

We kindly invite you to view our extensive catalog list at:
http://www.kessinger.net

PRINTED IN GREAT BRITAIN.
CHISWICK PRESS : CHARLES WHITTINGHAM AND GRIGGS (PRINTERS), LTD.
TOOKS COURT, CHANCERY LANE, LONDON.

CONTENTS

FOREWORD

RUDOLF STEINER, the teacher, guide, and friend, is no longer among the living on the Earth. A severe illness, beginning in sheer physical exhaustion, tore him away. In the very midst of his work he had to lie down on the bed of sickness. The powers he had devoted so copiously, so unstintingly, to the work of the Anthroposophical Society no longer sufficed to overcome his own illness. With untold grief and pain, all those who loved and honoured him had to stand by and witness how he who was loved by so many, who had been able to help so many others, had to allow Fate to take its appointed course when his own illness came, well knowing that higher powers were guiding these events.

In this small volume the fruits of our united work are recorded.

The teaching of Anthroposophy—for Medical Science a veritable mine of inspiration—I, as a Doctor, was able to confirm without reserve. I found in it a fount of wisdom from which it was possible untiringly to draw, and which was able to solve and illumine many a problem as yet unsolved in Medicine. Thus there arose between Rudolf Steiner and myself a living co-operation in the field of medical discovery. This co-operation, especially in the last two years, was deepened till the united authorship of a book became a possibility and an achievement. It had always been Rudolf Steiner's endeavour—and in this I could meet him with fullest sympathy of understanding—to renew the life of the ancient Mysteries and cause it to flow once more into the sphere of Medicine. From time immemorial, the Mysteries were most intimately united with the art of healing, and the attainment of spiritual knowledge was brought into connection with the healing of the sick. We had no thought, after the style of quacks and dilettanti, of underrating the scientific Medicine of our time. We recognized it fully. Our aim was to supplement the science already in existence by the illumination that can flow, from a true knowledge of the Spirit, towards a living grasp of the processes of illness and of healing. Needless to say, our purpose was to bring into new life, not the instinctive habit of the soul which still existed in the Mysteries of ancient time, but a method of research corresponding to the fully evolved consciousness of modern man, which can be lifted into spiritual regions.

Thus the first beginnings of our work were made. In the Clinical and Therapeutic Institute founded by myself at Arlesheim, in Switzerland, a basis was given in Practice for the Theories set forth in this book. And we endeavoured to unfold new ways in the art of healing to those who were seeking, in the sense here indicated, for a widening of their medical knowledge.

We had intended to follow up this small volume with further productions of our united work. This, alas, was no longer possible. It is, however, still my purpose, from the many notes and fruitful indications I received, to publish a second volume and possibly a third. As to this first volume, the manuscript of which was corrected with inner joy and satisfaction by Rudolf Steiner only three days before his death, may it find its way to those for whom it is intended—those who are striving to reach out from life's deep riddles to an understanding of life in its true greatness and glory.

ITA WEGMAN

Arlesheim-Dornach
September 1925.

Fundamentals of Therapy

CHAPTER I

TRUE KNOWLEDGE OF THE HUMAN BEING AS A FOUNDATION FOR THE ART OF MEDICINE

THIS book will indicate new possibilities for the science and art of Medicine. The reader must, however, be prepared to enter into the points of view which guided us when the medical conceptions here described came into being. If he cannot do so, he will not be in a position to form a proper judgment of what is brought forward in these pages.

There is no question of opposition to the Medicine that works with the recognized scientific methods of to-day. The latter, in its principles, is fully recognized by us; and we hold that what we have to give should be used in medical practice by those alone who are in the position of fully qualified doctors in accordance with these recognized principles.

On the other hand, to all that can be known about the human being with the methods that are recognized to-day, we add a further knowledge, whose discoveries are made by different methods. And out of this extended knowledge of the World and Man, we find ourselves compelled to work for an extension of the art of Medicine.

Fundamentally speaking, the recognized Medicine of to-day can offer no objection to what we have to say, seeing that we on our side do not deny its principles. He alone could reject our efforts *a priori*, who would require us not only to affirm his science but to adduce no further knowledge extending beyond the limits of his own.

In the Anthroposophy founded by Rudolf Steiner we see this extension of our knowledge of the World and Man. To the knowledge of the *physical* man, which is alone accessible to the natural-scientific methods of to-day, Anthroposophy adds that of the *spiritual* man. Nor does it merely proceed by a process of reflective thought from knowledge of the Physical to knowledge of the Spiritual. For on such a path, when all is said, one only finds oneself face to face with hypotheses more or less well conceived—hypotheses of which no one can prove that there is aught in reality to correspond to them.

Anthroposophy, before making any statements

2

about the Spiritual, evolves and elaborates the methods which give it the right to do so. Some insight will be gained into the nature of these methods if the following be considered: All the results of the accepted Science of our time are derived in the last resort from the impressions of the human senses. For to whatever degree, in experiment or in observation with the help of instruments, man may extend the sphere of what is yielded by his senses, nothing *in essence* new is added by these means to his experience of that world in which the senses place him.

But his thinking too, inasmuch as he applies it in his researches of the physical world, adds nothing new to what is given through the senses. In thinking he associates, analyses the sense-impressions, and so forth, in order to reach the laws (the Laws of Nature); yet the man who researches into this world must say to himself: " This thinking, as it wells up from within me, adds nothing real to what is already real in the world of sense."

Now all this at once becomes different if we no longer stop short at the thinking activity which is yielded, to begin with, by ordinary life and education. This thinking can be strengthened, vitalized within itself. We place some simple, easily encompassed thought in the centre of consciousness and, to the exclusion of all other thoughts, concentrate all the power of the soul on the one conception. Then, as a muscle grows strong when exerted again and again in the direction of the same force, our force of soul grows strong when exercised in this way with respect to that sphere of existence which otherwise holds sway in Thought. It should again be emphasized that these exercises must be based on simple, easily encompassed thoughts. For in carrying out the exercises the soul must not be exposed to any kind of influences from the unconscious or the semi-conscious. (Here we can but indicate the principle; a fuller description, and directions showing how such exercises should be done in individual cases, will be found in Rudolf Steiner's books, *Knowledge of the Higher Worlds and its Attainment, An Outline of Occult Science*, and other works in Anthroposophy.)

It is easy to make objection: that anyone who thus gives himself up with all his might to certain thoughts placed in the focus of his consciousness will thereby expose himself to all manner of auto-suggestion and the like, and that he will simply enter a realm of phantasy. But Anthroposophy shows how the exercises should be done from the outset, so that the objection loses its validity. It shows the way to advance within the sphere of consciousness, step by step and fully wide-awake in carrying out the exercises, as in the solving of an arithmetical or geometrical problem. At no point in solving a problem of Arithmetic or Geometry can our consciousness slide into unconscious regions; nor can it do so during the practices here indicated, provided always that the anthroposophical directions are properly observed.

In the course of such training we attain a strengthening of the *force of thought* of which we had not the remotest idea before. Like a new content of our human being we feel the force of thought holding sway within us. And with this new content of our own human being, there is revealed at the same time a World-content which, though we might perhaps have divined its existence, was unknown to us by experience till now.

If in a moment's introspection we consider our everyday activity of thought, we find that the thoughts are pale and shadow-like beside the impressions that our senses give us. What we perceive in the now strengthened force of thought is not pale or shadow-like by any means. It is full of inner content, vividly real and graphic; it is, indeed, of a reality far more intense than the contents of our sense-impressions.

A new world begins to dawn for the man who has thus enhanced the force of his perceptive faculty. He, who till now was only able to perceive in the world of the senses, learns to perceive in this new world; and as he does so he discovers that all the Laws of Nature known to him before hold good in the physical world only. It is of the essence of the world he has now entered, that its laws are different, nay, the very opposite of those of the physical world. In this world, for instance, the law of the force of attraction of the Earth does not hold good. On the contrary, another force emerges, working not from the centre of the Earth outward, but inversely. Its direction is from the circumference of the Universe towards the centre of the Earth. And so it is, in like manner, with the other forces of the physical world.

The faculty of man to perceive in this world, attainable as it is by exercise and training, is called in Anthroposophy the " Imaginative " faculty of knowledge. " Imaginative "—not that we have to do with " fancies " or imaginations in that sense; the word is used because the content of consciousness is filled with living pictures, instead of the shadows of thought.

In sense-perception we feel, as an immediate experience, that we are in a world of reality, and so we do in the activity of soul which is here called " Imaginative Knowledge." The world to

6

which this knowledge relates is called in Anthroposophy the "etheric" world. This is not to suggest the hypothetical ether of modern physics; it is something really *seen* in the Spirit. The name "etheric" is given to it in keeping with older, instinctive and dream-like, conceptions of that world. By the side of what can now be known with full clarity, those old conceptions no longer have a scientific value; but if we wish to designate a thing we have to choose some name.

Within the etheric world an etheric bodily nature of man is perceptible, existing in addition to the physical bodily nature.

This "etheric body" is to be found in its essential nature in the plant-world also. Plants, too, have their etheric body. In point of fact the physical laws only hold good for the world of lifeless mineral nature.

The plant-world is possible on Earth through the fact that there are substances in the earthly realm which do not remain enclosed within, or limited to, the physical laws. These substances can lay aside the whole complex of physical law and assume an opposite manner of working. The physical laws work, as it were, streaming outward from the Earth; the etheric, streaming toward the Earth from all directions of the World-circumference. Man cannot understand how the plant-world comes into being, till he sees in it the inter-play of the Earthly and physical with the Cosmic and " ethereal."

So it is with the etheric body of man himself. Through the etheric body something is taking place in man, which is not a straightforward continuation of the laws and workings of the physical body's forces, but rests on quite a different foundation. In effect the physical substances, as they pour into the etheric realm, divest themselves to begin with of their physical forces.

The forces that hold sway in the etheric body are active at the beginning of man's life on Earth, and most distinctly during the embryo period; they are the forces of growth and formative development. A portion of them, emancipated in the further course of earthly life from this formative activity, then becomes the force of thought. They are the forces which bring forth, for the ordinary consciousness, the shadow-like world of man's thoughts.

It is of the utmost importance to know that the ordinary thought-forces of man are the refined forces of bodily growth and formation. In the forming and growing of the human body, a Spiritual manifests itself. For it appears as such in the further course of life, in the spiritual force of thought.

8

The force of thought is but a part of the human force of growth and formation that works and weaves in the etheric. The other part remains true to the purpose it fulfils in the beginning of man's life. But the human being continues to evolve even when his formation and growth have reached an advanced stage—when they are to a certain degree complete. It is due to this alone that the etheric spiritual force, which lives and moves in the organic nature of the body, is able to emerge in later life as the force of thought.

Thus the formative (or plastic) force, appearing from the one side in the soul-content of our Thought, is revealed to the " imaginative " spiritual vision from the other side as an etheric-spiritual reality.

We may now follow the substantial nature of the earthly substances where they enter the etheric process, and we find: Wherever they do so the earthly substances themselves assume a form of being which estranges them from the physical nature. And while they are thus estranged, they enter into a world where the Spiritual comes to meet them, transforming them into its own being.

This way of ascending to the etherically living nature of man is a very different thing from the unscientific postulation of a " vital force " which was customary even to the middle of the nineteenth century in order to explain the living body. Here it is a question of the actual *seeing*—that is to say, the spiritual perception of a reality which is present, no less than the physical body, in man and in all living creatures. To reach this sight of the etheric we do not merely think on vaguely with the ordinary kind of thought; nor do we " think out " another world by dint of fancy. We extend the human powers of cognition by an exact and scientific process; and the straightforward result of this extension is to gain experience of an extended world.

The exercises leading to higher powers of perception can be carried farther. Just as we exert a heightened force in concentrating on thoughts placed deliberately in the centre of our consciousness, so we can apply a greater force again to suppress the Imaginations—the pictures of a spiritual-etheric reality—attained by the former process. We then reach a condition of completely emptied consciousness. We are awake and aware, but our awareness to begin with has no content. (Further details are to be found in the above-mentioned books.)

But this awareness without content does not remain so. Our consciousness, emptied as it is of any physical or even etherically pictorial impressions, becomes filled with a content that pours into it from a real spiritual world, even as the impressions from the physical world pour into the physical senses.

By Imaginative Knowledge we learn to know a second member of the human being; by the emptied consciousness becoming filled with spiritual content we learn to know a third. Anthroposophy calls the power of knowledge that comes about in this way " Knowledge by Inspiration." (The reader should not let these terms offend him. They are borrowed from the instinctive ways of looking into spiritual worlds which belonged to more primitive ages, but the sense in which they are here used is stated scientifically.) The world to which man gains entry by " Inspiration " is called in Anthroposophy the " astral world."

Speaking, in the manner here explained, of an " etheric world," we refer to the influences that work from the circumference of the Universe towards the Earth. When we go on to speak of the " astral world," we proceed, according to the perceptions of Inspired Consciousness, from the influences from the World-circumference to the spiritual Beings who reveal themselves in these influences—just as the materials of the Earth reveal their nature in the forces that go outward from the Earth. We speak of definite spiritual

Beings working from the universal spaces, just as we speak of the stars and constellations when with the eye of sense we watch the heavens at night-time. Hence the expression " astral world." In the astral world man bears the third member of his human nature, namely his astral body.

Into the astral body, too, the substantial natures of the Earth must flow. They are thereby estranged still more from their physical nature. Man, as we saw, has the etheric body in common with the world of plants; he has the astral body in common with the world of animals.

The essentially human being, whereby man is raised above and beyond the animal creation, is known by a form of knowledge still higher than Inspiration. At this point Anthroposophy speaks of Intuition. In Inspiration a World of spiritual Beings is revealed; in the act of knowledge which we here call Intuition, the relation of the human being to that World grows more intimate. He now brings to fullest consciousness within him that which is purely Spiritual, and of which he knows—immediately in the conscious experience of it—that it has nothing to do with any experience conveyed through the bodily nature. He transplants himself into a new life which can only be described as a life of the human Spirit among other Spirit-Beings. In Inspiration the spiritual

Beings of the World reveal themselves; through Intuition we ourselves *live with* the Beings.[1]

In this way we come to recognize the fourth member of the human being—the essential " I " or " Ego." Once again we become aware how the substantial nature of the Earth, in entering the life and being of the " Ego," is estranged still more from its physical form of existence. The nature which it here assumes—the " organization of the Ego "—is, to begin with, that form of earthly substance in which the latter is farthest estranged from its earthly, physical character.

In the human organization what we thus learn to know as the " astral body " and " Ego " is not bound to the physical body in the same way as is the etheric body. Inspiration and Intuition show how in sleep the astral body and the Ego separate from the physical and etheric; it is only in the waking state that there is the full mutual permeation of the four members to form the single and united nature of man.

[1] *Note by Translator.* Dr. Steiner uses the identical words —*Imagination, Inspiration, Intuition*—in the German original of this and other anthroposophical works. Occurring as they do more frequently in English in the colloquial meanings of ordinary speech, we distinguish them here by a capital letter when used in the technical sense of Anthroposophy to denote the higher powers of cognition.

In sleep the physical and the etheric human body are left behind in the physical and etheric world. But they are not in the same position as the physical and etheric body of a plant or plant-like being. For they bear within them the after-influences of the astral and the Ego-nature. Indeed, the moment they would no longer bear these influences within them, the human being must awaken. A human physical body must never be subject to the merely physical, nor a human etheric body to the mere etheric influences. Under such influences alone they would disintegrate.

Yet another thing is revealed by Inspiration and Intuition. The physical substantial natures, as they pass on to live and move in the etheric, are carried to a higher form of organization. And *Life* itself depends upon the fact that the organic body, freed from a mere earthly form of existence, is built up by forces working inward from the Universe beyond the Earth. But while this *upbuilding* process leads to *Life*, it does not lead to *Consciousness* nor to *Self-Consciousness*. The astral body must build up its own organization within the physical and the etheric, and for the " Ego-organization " the Ego must do the same. But this upbuilding process is not accompanied by any conscious unfolding of the soul's life. For the latter to ensue, the upbuilding process must be opposed by one of *demolition*. The astral body builds up its organs; it destroys them again, and in so doing enables the activity of Feeling to unfold in consciousness of soul. The Ego builds up its "Ego-organization"; it destroys it again, when in Self-consciousness the activity of Will becomes effective.

Thus the Spirit (the mental life) unfolds in human nature, not on the basis of constructive activities of substance, but of destructive. At whatsoever point in man the Spirit is to work, material substance must withdraw from its activity.

Even the rise of Thought in the etheric body rests not on a further development but on a destruction of etheric life and being. *Conscious* thinking takes place, not in the actual processes of growth and formation, but in processes of deformation—fading, dying processes—which are continually interwoven with the etheric life.

In the act of conscious thinking, the thoughts loose themselves from bodily formation to emerge as formations in the soul, in the conscious experience of man.

With the foundation of such a knowledge of man, we can now observe the human being, and we become aware that the nature of the whole man, or of any single organ, is only seen with clarity by recognizing how the physical, the etheric, the astral body, and the Ego are at work there.

There are organs in which the Ego is paramountly active; in others the Ego works but little, and the physical organization is predominant.

The healthy human nature can only be understood by recognizing how the higher members of man's being take possession of the earthly substance, compelling it into their service. In this connection we must also recognize how the earthly substance becomes transformed when it enters the sphere of action of the higher members. And so it is with the man diseased. We only understand him when we perceive how the organism as a whole, or a certain organ or series of organs, become affected when the mode of action of the higher members falls into irregularity. We shall only be able to think of remedies when we evolve a knowledge of how some earthly substance or earthly process is related to the Etheric, to the Astral, to the Ego. For only then, by introducing an earthly substance to the human body or by treatment with an earthly process of activity, shall we be able to achieve the desired result, enabling the higher members of the human being to unfold again unhindered, or providing the earthly substance of the body—in the added medicament or treatment—with the assistance it may need, to bring it into the path where it becomes a basis for the earthly working of the Spiritual.

Man is what he is by virtue of body, etheric body, soul (aſtral body), and Ego (Spirit). He muſt, in health, be seen and underſtood from the aspeɕt of these his members; in disease he muſt be observed in the diſturbance of their equilibrium; and for his healing we muſt find the remedies that can reſtore the balance.

A medical conception built on such foundations is to be indicated in these pages.

CHAPTER II

WHY MAN IS SUBJECT TO ILLNESS

ANYONE who reflects on the fact that the human being can be diseased, will find himself involved in a paradox which he cannot avoid if he wishes to think purely on the lines of Natural Science. He will have to assume to begin with that this paradox lies in the very nature of existence. For, outwardly considered, whatever takes place in the process of disease is a process of Nature. But that which replaces it in health is also a process of Nature.

In the first place, the processes of Nature are known to us only by observation of the world external to Man, and of Man himself inasmuch as we set to work observing him in just the same way as we observe external Nature. In doing so, we conceive him as a piece of Nature. We conceive that the processes going on within him, however complicated, are of the same kind as the processes we can observe outside him—the outer processes of Nature.

Here, however, a question emerges which is quite unanswerable from this point of view. How do there arise in Man (not to speak, at this point, of the animal) processes of Nature which run counter to the healthy ones?

The healthy human body seems to be intelligible as a piece of Nature; the diseased does not. It must, therefore, be intelligible in itself, by virtue of something which it does not receive from Nature.

It is commonly thought that the mental and spiritual in Man has for its physical foundation a complicated process of Nature—a further elaboration of the processes we find outside him. But let us observe after all whether the continuation of any process of Nature, taking its place in the healthy human body, ever does call forth conscious mental or spiritual experience as such. The reverse is the case. The conscious life of the Spirit is extinguished when the process of Nature is continued in a straightforward line. This is what happens in sleep; it happens, too, in faintness.

Consider on the other hand how the conscious mental life is sharpened when an organ becomes diseased. Pain ensues, or—at the least—discomfort and displeasure. The sentient life of Feeling receives a content which it lacks in ordinary

life, and the life of Will is impaired. The movement of a limb, which takes place as a matter of
course in the healthy state, can no longer be
accomplished properly; the pain or discomfort
hinders and opposes it.

Observe now the transition from the painful
movement of a limb to its paralysis. In the movement accompanied by pain we have the initial
stages of a movement paralysed. The actively
Spiritual takes hold of the body. In the healthy
condition it reveals itself to begin with in the life
of thought or ideation. We actuate a certain idea,
and the movement of a limb ensues. We do not
enter consciously with the idea into the organic
processes which culminate in the movement.
The idea dives down into the unconscious.
Between the idea and the movement an act of
feeling intervenes; but this—in the healthy condition—works in the soul only, it does not attach
itself distinctly to any bodily organic process.
In disease, however, it is different. The feeling,
experienced in health as a thing distinct and apart,
unites with the physical organization in the
conscious experience of illness.

The healthy processes of feeling and the conscious experience of illness thus appear in their
relationship. Something must be there, which,
when the body is in health, is less intensely united

with it than when it is diseased. To spiritual perception this " something " is revealed to be the astral body. The astral body is a super-sensible organization within that which the senses can perceive. If it takes hold of an organ but loosely, it leads to an inner experience of soul—an experience which subsists in itself and is not felt to be in connection with the body. If, on the other hand, the astral body takes hold of an organ strongly or intensely, it leads to the consciousness of illness. One of the forms of illness must indeed be conceived as an abnormal seizure of the organ-ism by the astral body. This form of illness causes the Spiritual Man to dive down into his body more deeply than is the case in health.

Now Thinking, too, has its physical foundation in the body. In health however, it is still more loosely connected, still freer of the bodily founda-tion, than the life of feeling. Spiritual perception finds beside the astral body a special Ego-organiza-tion which lives and expresses itself with freedom of soul in thought. If with this Ego-organization man takes intense hold of his bodily nature, the ensuing condition makes his observation of his own organism similar to that of the external world. That is to say: When he observes a thing or process of the outer world, the thought in man and the object observed are not in living mutual interplay, but independent of one another. In a human limb this condition only takes place when it is paralysed. It then becomes a part of the external world. The Ego-organization is no longer loosely united with the limb, as when in health it can unite with it in the act of movement and withdraw again at once. It dives down permanently into the limb and is no longer able to withdraw itself.

Here again the processes of the healthy movement of a limb and of paralysis stand side by side in their relationship. Nay more, we recognize distinctly: The healthy act of movement is a paralysis in its initial stages—a paralysis which is arrested as soon as it begins.

We must see the very essence of illness in this intensive union of the astral body or Ego-organization with the physical organism. But this union is only an intensification of that which exists more loosely in a state of health. Even the normal way in which the astral and Ego-organization take hold of the human body, is related not to the healthy processes of life, but to the diseased. Wherever the soul and Spirit are at work, they annul the ordinary functioning of the body, transforming it into its opposite. In so doing they bring the body into a line of action where illness tends to set in.

In normal life this is regulated directly it arises by a process of self-healing.

A certain form of illness occurs when the Spiritual, or the soul, pushes its way forward too far into the organism, with the result that the self-healing process can either not take place at all or is too slow.

In the faculties of soul and Spirit, therefore, we have to seek the causes of disease. Healing must then consist in loosening this element of soul or Spirit from the physical organization.

This is the one kind of disease. There is another. The Ego-organization and the astral body may be prevented from reaching even that looser union with the bodily nature which is conditioned, in ordinary life, by the independent activities of Feeling, Thought, and Will. Then, in the organs or processes which the soul and Spirit are thus unable to approach, there will be a continuation of the healthy processes beyond the measure that is right for the organism as a whole. But spiritual perception shows that in such a case the physical organism does not merely carry out the lifeless processes of external Nature. For the physical organism is permeated by an etheric. The physical organism alone could never call forth a process of self-healing; it is in the etheric organism that this process is kindled. We are thus led to recognize health as that condition which has its origin in the etheric. Healing must therefore consist in a treatment of the etheric organism.[1]

[1] The point of this will best be understood by carefully comparing the contents of this Second Chapter with what was said above, in the First.

CHAPTER III

THE PHENOMENA OF LIFE

WE cannot come to understand the human organism, in health or in disease, if we conceive that the characteristic reactions of any substance, absorbed in the process of nourishment, are simply continued from external Nature into the inner parts of the body. Within the human body it is not a question of continuing, but, on the contrary, of overcoming the reactions observable in the substance while outside the body.

The illusion that the substances of the outer world simply continue to work of their own nature in the body, is due to the fact that to the ordinary chemical conception of to-day it appears to be so. Following the researches of this Chemistry, the scientist gives himself up to the belief that Hydrogen, for instance, is present in the body in the same form as in external Nature, since it occurs, first in the substances consumed as food and drink, and then in the products of excretion: air, sweat, urine, fæces, or in secretions, such as bile.

The scientist of to-day feels no necessity to ask what happens in the organism to that which appears as Hydrogen before its entry into and after its exit from the same. Outside the organism it appears as Hydrogen. He does not ask: What does it undergo while it is within the living body?

When however we do raise this question, we are at once impelled to turn our attention to the difference between the organism waking and asleep. When the organism is asleep, its substantial nature provides no basis for the unfolding of conscious or self-conscious experience. But it still provides a basis for the unfolding of life. In this respect the sleeping organism is distinguished from the dead, for the substantial basis of the latter is no longer one of life. And so long as we merely see the distinction in a different constitution or arrangement of substances as between the living organism and the dead, we shall not really progress in our understanding of the matter.

It is wellnigh half a century since the eminent physiologist, Du Bois Reymond, pointed out that consciousness can and will never be explained by the reactions of material substance. Never, he declared, shall we understand why it should not be a matter of indifference to so many atoms of Carbon, Oxygen, Hydrogen, and Nitrogen what their relative position is or was or will become, or why by these their changes of position, they should bring forth in Man the sensations, " I see red," " I smell the scent of roses." Such being the case, Du Bois Reymond contended, natural-scientific thought can never explain the waking human being, filled as he is with sensations; it can only explain the sleeping man.

Yet in this hope too he gave himself up to an illusion. He believed that the phenomena of life, though not of consciousness, would be intelligible as an outcome of the reactions of material substance. But, in reality, we must say of the phenomena of life, as he said of those of consciousness: Why should it occur to so many atoms of Carbon, Oxygen, Hydrogen, and Nitrogen to bring forth —by the manner of their present, past, or future relative positions—the phenomenon of life?

Observation shows, after all, that the phenomena of life have an altogether different orientation from those that run their course within the lifeless realm. Of the latter we shall be able to say, they reveal that they are subject to forces radiating outward from the essence of material substance. These forces radiate from the—relative—centre to the periphery. But in the phenomena of life, the material substance appears subject to forces working from without inward—towards the relative centre. Passing on into the sphere of life, the substance must withdraw itself from the forces raying outward and subject itself to those that radiate inward.

Now it is to the Earth that every earthly substance, or earthly process, owes its forces of the kind that radiate outward. It has these forces in common with the Earth. It is, indeed, only as a constituent of the Earth-body that any substance has the nature which Chemistry discovers in it. And when it comes to life, it must cease to be a mere portion of the Earth; it leaves its community with the Earth and is gathered up into the forces that ray inward to the Earth from all sides—from beyond the earthly realm. Whenever we see a substance or process unfold in forms of life, we must conceive it to be withdrawing from the forces that work upon it as from the centre of the Earth, and entering the domain of others, which have, not a centre, but a periphery.

From all sides they work, these forces, striving as if towards the central point of the Earth. They would tear asunder the substantial nature of the earthly realm, dissolve it into complete formlessness, were it not for the Heavenly bodies beyond the Earth which mingle their influences in the field of these forces and modify the dissolving process. In the plant we can observe what happens. In plants, the substances of the earth are lifted out of the domain of earthly influences; they tend towards the formless. But this transition to the formless is modified by the influences of the Sun and similar effects from universal space. When these are no longer working, or when they are working differently, as in the night, then in the substances the forces which they have from their community with Earth begin to stir once more. From the working together of earthly forces and cosmic, the plant-nature arises. And if we comprise in the term "Physical" the domain of all those forces and reactions which the substances unfold under the Earth's influence, we shall have to designate the entirely different forces which radiate—not outward from the Earth—but in towards it, by a name in which this different character must find expression. Here we come from another aspect to that element in the organization of Man which was indicated from one aspect in the former chapter. In harmony with an older usage—which has fallen into confusion under the modern purely physical way of thinking—we have agreed to denote this part of the human organism as the "Etheric." Thus, we shall have to say: In the plant-like nature, inasmuch as it appears alive, the Etheric is holding sway.

In Man too, inasmuch as he is a living being, the same etheric principle holds sway. Nevertheless, even with respect to the mere phenomena of life, an important difference is apparent in his nature as against the plant's. For the plant lets the Physical hold sway within it when the Etheric from the Cosmic spaces is no longer unfolding its influence, as is the case when at night-time the Sun-ether ceases to work. The human being, on the other hand, only lets the Physical hold sway within his body when death takes place. In sleep, though the phenomena of consciousness and self-consciousness vanish away, the phenomena of life remain, even when the Sun-ether is no longer working in the Cosmic spaces. Perpetually, throughout its life, the plant is receiving into itself the Ether-forces as they ray in towards the Earth. Man, however, carries them within himself in an individualized way, even from the embryonic period of his existence. Man, during his life, takes *out of himself* what the plant receives continually from the Universe. In effect, he received it for his further development already in the mother's womb. A force whose proper nature is originally cosmic—destined to pour its influences in towards the Earth—pours forth from lung or liver. It has undergone a metamorphosis of its direction.

Thus we shall have to say: Man bears the Etheric within him in an individualized form.

As he carries the Physical in the individualized form of his physical body and its organs, so too with the Etheric. He has his own special etheric body, as he has the physical. In sleep, this etheric body remains united with the physical and gives it life; it only separates from it in death.

CHAPTER IV

NATURE OF THE SENTIENT ORGANISM

THE plant form and plant organization are an exclusive product of the two domains of forces: those radiating outward from the Earth and in towards it. The animal and human are not exclusively so. The leaf of a plant stands under the influence of these two domains of forces to the exclusion of all others; the lung of an animal is subject to the same influences, but not exclusively. For the leaf, all the formative creative forces lie within the two domains, while for the lung there are other formative forces outside them. This applies both to the formative forces which give the outward shape, and to those that regulate the inner movements of the substances, giving them a definite direction, combining them or separating them.

Of the substances absorbed into the plant we can say indeed, that, owing to their entry into the domain of forces raying in towards the Earth, it does not remain a matter of indifference to them whether they are alive or not. They are lifeless even within the plant when the forces of the World-circumference are not working on them; they enter into life when they come under the influence of these forces.

But to the plant substance, even when alive, the past, present, or future relative position of its members is a matter of indifference so far as any action of their own is concerned. They abandon themselves to the action of the external forces—those radiating out and inward. The animal substance comes to action in ways that are independent of these forces. It moves within the organism—or the whole organism moves—in such a way that the movements do not follow exclusively the outpouring and inpouring forces. The animal configuration arises independently of the domains of forces radiating outward from and in towards the Earth.

In the plant, the play of forces here described gives rise to an alternation between the conditions of being connected and disconnected—if we may borrow these expressions—with the current of the forces that pour in from the periphery. The single being of the plant thus falls into two parts. The one tends to life and is wholly under the domain of the World-circumference; these are the springing, sprouting organs, the growing and blossom-

D

ing. The other inclines towards the lifeless, it stays in the domain of the forces raying outward from the Earth. This part comprises all that hardens the growth, provides a firm support for life, and so on. Between the two parts, life is for ever being kindled and extinguished, and when the plant dies, it is simply that the outpouring forces gain the upper hand over the inpouring.

Now, in the animal, a part of the substantial nature is drawn right out of the domain of these two kinds of forces. Another partition is thus brought about, over and above what we found in the plant. Organic formations arise which stay within the domain of the two kinds of forces, but others too come into being, which are lifted out of this domain. Between these two formations, mutual interactions take place, and in these interactions we have the real cause enabling the animal substance to become a vehicle of sentient life. Another consequence is the difference, both in outward appearance and inner constitution, as between the animal substance and the plant.

Thus in the animal organism we have a domain of forces independent of those radiating outward from and inward to the Earth. Beside the physical and the etheric, there is in fact the astral domain of forces, of which we have already spoken from another point of view. One need not take offence

34

at the term " astral." The outpouring forces are the earthly ones; the inpouring are those of the World-circumference about the Earth. In the " astral," something is present of a higher order than these two kinds of forces. This higher presence first makes of the Earth itself a heavenly body within the Universe—a " Star " or *Astrum*. Through the physical forces the Earth separates itself from the Universe; through the etheric it subjects itself to the influence of the Universe upon it. With the " astral " forces it becomes, within the Universe, an independent Individuality.

In the animal organism, the " astral " principle is an independent, self-contained organization like the physical and the etheric. We can therefore speak of this organization as an " astral body."

The whole animal organization is only intelligible by studying the mutual relationships between the physical, the etheric, and the astral body. For all three are present, independently, as its members. Not only so, each of the three is different from anything that exists outside, by way of lifeless (mineral) bodies or living bodies of a plant-like nature.

True, the animal physical organism can be spoken of as lifeless; yet it is different from the lifeless nature of the mineral. For it is first estranged by the etheric and the astral organism

from the mineral nature; and then, by a with-
drawal of etheric and astral forces, it is returned to
the lifeless realm. It is an entity in which the
mineral forces—those that work in the Earth-
domain alone—can only act destructively. This
physical body can serve the animal organization
as a whole, only so long as the etheric and astral
maintain the upper hand over the destructive
intervention of the mineral forces.

The animal etheric organization is living, like
that of the plant—but not in the same manner.
By the astral forces, the life has been brought into
a condition foreign to itself; it has in fact been
torn away from the forces raying in towards the
Earth and then returned once more to their domain.
The etheric organism is an entity in which the
plant-like forces have an existence too dull and
stupid for the animal nature. Only through the
astral forces continually lighting up its manner of
activity can it serve the animal organism as a whole.
If the activities of the etheric gain the upper hand,
sleep ensues; if the astral organism becomes predominant, the creature is awake.

Sleeping and Waking: Neither the one nor the
other must exceed a certain limit in its mode of
action. If this were to happen in the case of
Sleep, the plant-nature in the organism as a whole
would incline towards the mineral; there would

arise a morbid condition—a hypertrophy of the plant-nature. And if it happened in the case of Waking, the plant-nature would become entirely estranged from the mineral and the latter would assume forms within the organism belonging not to it, but to the external, inorganic, lifeless sphere. It would be a morbid condition by hypertrophy of the mineral nature.

Into all the three organisms—physical, etheric, and astral—physical substance penetrates from outside. Each of the three in its own way must overcome the special nature of the physical. A threefold organization is thus brought into being.

The physical organism produces organs which have gone through the etheric and astral organizations and are on the way back again to the purely physical domain. They cannot altogether have arrived there, for this would mean death to the whole body.

The etheric organism produces organs which have passed through the astral organization but are striving ever and again to withdraw from it. They have in them the force that inclines to the dull stupor of Sleep; they tend to unfold a purely vegetative life.

The astral organism produces organs which estrange, or put away from them, the vegetative life. Yet they can only exist if this vegetative life takes hold of them again and again. Having no relationship either with the outpouring or with the inpouring forces of the Earth, they would fall out of the earthly realm altogether if it did not again and again take hold of them. In these organs, a rhythmic interplay of the animal and plant-like natures must take place. This determines the alternating states of Sleeping and Waking. In Sleep, the organs of the astral forces, too, are in the dull stupor of a plant-like life. They then have no active influence on the etheric and physical, which are thus entirely abandoned to the domains of forces pouring in towards and outward from the Earth.

CHAPTER V

PLANT, ANIMAL, AND MAN

IN the astral body the animal form arises: outwardly the form as a whole, inwardly the formation of the organs. The sentient animal substance is, then, an outcome of the form-giving activity of the astral body. Where this process of formation is carried to its conclusion, the animal nature is produced.

In man it is not carried to its conclusion. At a certain point on its way it is hindered and arrested.

In the plant we have material substance transformed by the forces radiating in towards the Earth. This is the living substance, and it is continually interacting with the lifeless. We must conceive that in the plant, living substance is perpetually being separated out of the lifeless. In the living substance, the plant form then becomes apparent, as a product of the forces raying in towards the Earth. Thus we have a single stream of substance: lifeless substance being transformed into living, living into lifeless. In this stream the organs of the plant come into being.

In the animal the sentient substance comes forth from the living, as in the plant the living from the lifeless. Thus there is a twofold stream of substance. The life is not carried to the point of finished living form within the etheric realm. It is kept in flow, and into the flowing life the astral organism inserts its principle of form.

In man, this latter process, too, is kept in flow. The sentient substance is drawn into the realm of a still further organization, which we can call the " organization of the Ego." Thus the sentient substance is transformed once more and a three-fold stream of substance is produced. In this the human form—inwardly no less than outwardly—arises, and becomes the bearer of self-conscious spiritual life. Down to the smallest particle of his substance, man in his form and configuration is a product of the organization of the Ego.

We can now trace these processes of formation in their substantial aspect. The transformation of substance from the one level to the next appears as a separating of the substance on the higher level from the lower, and a building of the form out of the substance thus " sublimated." Thus, in the plant: out of the lifeless substance the living is sublimated, and in the latter the etheric forces work, radiating in towards the Earth, creating the plant's form. To begin with there takes place, not a separation properly speaking, but an entire transformation of physical substance by the etheric forces. This however only happens in the creation of the seed. Here the transformation can be complete, because the seed is protected by the surrounding maternal envelope from the influences of the physical forces. But when the seed-formation is freed from the maternal organism, the working of forces in the plant divides into two members. On the one hand, the forming of substance strives into the realm of the etheric, while on the other hand it strives back again to physical formation. Thus there arise the members of the plant which are on the way of life and the others which incline to fall off and die. The latter then appear as the " excreted " members of the plant organism. The bark-formation of the tree is a characteristic example in which we may observe this excreting process.

In the animal the process of separation, both upward and downward, is twofold. There is, as it were, a twofold " sublimation " and a twofold " excretion." The plant-process of transformation, as we have seen, is not carried to a conclusion but kept in flow, and there is added to it the transformation of living substance into sentient. Sentient substance separates out of the merely living.

We have therefore, on the one hand, substance that is striving towards sentient existence, and on the other, substance that is striving away from it to the condition of mere life.

Now in an organism mutual interaction comes about as between all its members. Hence in the animal the excretion towards the lifeless realm—which in the plant approaches very nearly to the outer lifeless world, the mineral,—still remains far removed from mineral nature. In the bark-forming process of the plant, we see the forming of a substance which is already on the way to mineral nature and loosens itself from the plant-organism increasingly the more mineral it becomes. In the animal realm the same process appears in the excreted products of digestion, but these are farther removed from the mineral nature than the " excretions " of the plant.

In man a further stage is reached. There separates out, from the sentient substance, that which becomes the vehicle of the self-conscious Spirit. But a continual downward separation is also brought about, for in the process, substance is produced that strives towards the merely sentient faculty. Thus the animal nature is present within the human organism as a perpetual " excretion."

In the animal organism, in the waking state, the " sublimation " of sentient substance and its

42

creation into form, as well as the accompanying downward or " excretive " process, are under the influence of the astral activity. In man there is also the activity of the Ego-organism. In sleep the astral and the Ego-organism are not directly active; but the substance has been taken hold of by their activity and continues in it as though by inertia. A substance once shaped and permeated through and through by the workings of the astral and Ego-organizations, will go on working in their sense even during sleep, by force of inertia, as it were.

We cannot therefore speak of any merely vegetative action of the organism in the sleeping man. The astral and Ego-organizations work on in the substance that is formed under their influence, even in the state of sleep. The difference between sleeping and waking is not represented by an alternation of human and animal with physical and vegetative modes of action. The true fact is altogether different. In waking life the sentient substance and that which can act as a vehicle of the self-conscious Spirit are lifted out of the organism as a whole and placed in the service of the astral body and Ego-organization. The physical and etheric organism must then work in such a way that the outpouring and inpouring forces of the Earth are alone active within them.

In this mode of action they are taken hold of by the astral body and Ego-organization only from outside. In sleep on the other hand, they are taken hold of inwardly by the substances that come into existence under the influence of astral body and Ego-organization. While man is sleeping, and from the Universe as a whole only the forces radiating out of the Earth and in towards it work upon him, there are working upon him from within the substance-forces which the astral body and Ego-organization have prepared. If we call the sentient substance the *residue* of the astral body, and that which has arisen under the Ego-organization's influence its residue, then we may say: In the waking human organism the astral body and Ego-organization themselves are working, and in the sleeping human organism their substantial residues.

In waking life man lives in activities which bring him into connection with the outer world through his astral body and through his Ego-organization. In sleep his physical and etheric body live by what the residues of these two organizations in substance have become. A substance absorbed by man—like Oxygen in breathing—both in the sleeping and in the waking state, must therefore be distinguished as to its mode of action in the two conditions. By its own inherent nature,

44

the Oxygen absorbed from without has the effect not of awakening, but of putting man to sleep. In waking life the astral body battles perpetually against the soporific influence of the absorption of Oxygen. When the astral body suspends its work upon the physical, the Oxygen unfolds its proper nature and sends the man to sleep.

CHAPTER VI

BLOOD AND NERVE

THE activities of the several human organizations in relation to the organism as a whole are strikingly expressed in the formation of the blood and nerves. Where the foodstuffs absorbed into the body become progressively transformed in the process of blood-formation, this whole process stands under the influence of the Ego-organization. From the processes that take place in the tongue and palate, accompanied by conscious sensation, down to the unconscious and sub-conscious processes in the workings of pepsin, pancreatic juice, bile, etc., the Ego-organization is at work. Then the working of the Ego-organization withdraws to some extent, and in the further transformation of foodstuffs into the substance of blood the astral body is predominantly active. This goes on up to the point where, in the breathing process, the blood meets the air—that is to say, the oxygen. At this point the etheric body

46

carries out its main activity. In the carbonic acid that is on the point of being breathed out but has not yet left the body, we have a substance which is in the main only living—that is to say, it is neither sentient, nor dead. (Everything is alive that carries in it the activity of the etheric body.) The main quantity of this living carbonic acid leaves the organism, but a small proportion continues within the organism, working into the processes that have their centre in the head-organization. This portion shows a strong tendency to pass into the lifeless inorganic nature, but it does not become entirely lifeless.

The nervous system shows an opposite distribution. In the sympathetic nervous system which permeates the organs of digestion, the etheric body is paramountly holding sway. The nerve-organs with which we are here concerned are of their own nature merely living organs. The astral and Ego-organizations do not organize them from within but affect them only from outside. For this very reason the influence of the astral and Ego-organizations working in these nerve-organs is powerful. Passions and emotions have a deep and lasting effect upon the sympathetic nervous system; sorrow and anxiety will gradually ruin it.

The nervous system of the spinal cord, with its many ramifications, is the one in which the astral organization pre-eminently takes effect. Hence it is the vehicle of that in man which belongs to the soul-nature—namely the reflex processes—but not of that which takes place in the self-conscious Spirit, in the Ego.

It is the brain-nerves, properly speaking, which are subject to the Ego-organization. In these the activities of the etheric and astral organizations fall into the background.

We thus see three distinct regions arising in the organism as a whole. In a lower region, nerves permeated from within mainly by the action of the etheric organism work with a blood substance that is paramountly subject to the activity of the Ego-organization. In this region, during the embryonic and post-embryonic period of development, we have the starting-point for all organ-formations connected with the inner vitalization of the human body. In the formation of the embryo, this region, being weak as yet, is supplied with the formative and life-giving influences by the surrounding mother-organism. Then there is a middle region, where nerve-organs, influenced by the astral organization, are working with blood-processes which are likewise dependent on the astral and, in their upper parts, on the etheric. Here, in the early periods of development, there lies the starting-point for the formation of the organs that are

48

instrumental in the processes of outer and inner movement. This applies not only to the muscles for example, but to all organs which are causes of mobility, whether or not they be muscles in the proper sense. Finally there is an upper region, where nerves subject to the inner organizing activity of the Ego work with blood processes that have a strong tendency to pass into the lifeless mineral realm. Here lies the starting-point, during the early epoch of man's development, for the formation of the bones and everything else that serves the human body for organs of support.

We shall only understand the brain of man if we see in it a bone-forming tendency interrupted in its very first beginning. Nor shall we understand the bone-forming process until we recognize in it the working of the same impulses as in the brain. In the bone-formation, the brain-impulse is carried to its final conclusion and permeated from without by the impulses of the middle body, where astrally conditioned nerve-organs are working together with blood-substance etherically conditioned. In the bone-ash which remains over with its peculiar configuration when the bones are subjected to combustion, we see the creations of the uppermost region of the human organization; while, in the organic residue which is left behind when the bones are treated with dilute hydrochloric acid, we have the outcome of the impulses of the middle region.

The skeleton is the physical image of the Ego-organization. For in the bone-creating process the human organic substance, as it tends towards the lifeless mineral nature, submits entirely to the Ego-organization. In the brain on the other hand, the Ego is active as a spiritual being. Here its form-creating force—its power to work into the physical—is quite overwhelmed by the organizing activity of the Etheric, nay more, by the forces inherent in the Physical. The brain-formation is founded only to a slight extent on the Ego's organizing power, which here becomes submerged in the processes of Life and in the inherent workings of the Physical. Yet this is the very reason why the brain is the vehicle of the spiritual actions of the Ego. For, inasmuch as the organic and physical activities in the brain do not involve the Ego-organization, the latter is able to devote itself to its own entirely free activities. In the bony system of the skeleton, perfect though it is as a physical picture of the same, the Ego-organization exhausts itself in the act of organizing the physical, and as a spiritual activity nothing is left of it. Hence the processes in the bones are the most unconscious.

So long as it is in the body, the carbonic acid driven outward by the breathing process is still a living substance. It is taken hold of and driven outward by the astral activity that has its seat in the middle or spinal region of the nervous system. The portion of carbonic acid which goes with the metabolism towards the head is there brought into union with calcium, and thus receives a tendency to come into the sphere of action of the Ego-organization. The calcium carbonate is then driven on the way to bone-formation under the influence of the head-nerves, filled as they are from within by the Ego-organization with its impulses.

The substances myosin and myogen (paramyosinogen and myosinogen), produced out of the foodstuffs, tend to become deposited in the blood. They are substances astrally conditioned to begin with, and they stand in mutual interaction with the Sympathetic, which is organized from within by the etheric body. These albuminous substances are however also taken hold of, to some extent, by the action of the spinal nervous system which is under the influence of the astral body. They thus come into relation with the disintegration-products of albumen, with fats, sugar, and other substances similar to sugar. This enables them, under the influence of the spinal nervous system, to find their way into the process of muscle-formation.

51

CHAPTER VII

NATURE OF THE INFLUENCES OF HEALING

THE human organism as a whole is not a self-contained system of processes interlocked with one another. If it were so, it could not be a vehicle of soul and Spirit. In the substances of nerve and bone and in the processes of which they are a part, the human body is perpetually disintegrating, or entering upon the path of lifeless, mineral activities. In this way alone can it provide the soul and Spirit with a foundation of activity.

In the nervous tissues albuminous substance disintegrates; but in these tissues—unlike what happens in the egg and other organic forms—it is not built up again by coming into the domain of influences radiating in towards the Earth. It simply disintegrates; and the Ether-influences radiating in through the senses from the things and processes of the environment, as well as those that arise when the organs of movement are made use of, are thereby enabled to use the nerves as organs along which they are carried throughout the body.

In the nerves there are two kinds of processes: the disintegration of albumen [1] and the permeation of this disintegrating substance with flowing etheric substance, whose flow is started and stimulated by acids, salts, and materials of the character of phosphorus and sulphur. The equilibrium between the two processes is brought about by fats and water.

Seen in their essential nature, these are processes of disease which permeate the organism all the time. They must be balanced by no less continuous processes of healing.

Now the balance is brought about through the blood, which contains not only the processes that constitute growth and metabolism. In effect, we must also attribute to the blood a constant healing action by which the morbid processes in the nerves are opposed.

In the plasma and fibrinogen, the blood contains those forces which serve the growth and

Note by Translator. Here, and throughout the book, the word " albumen " is applied, not only to the albumens in the narrower sense, but to the whole class of the " proteins " (German *Eiweiss-Stoffe*—albuminous substances). We are aware that a different nomenclature has been adopted, since the year 1907, by English and American scientists; but for our purpose it seemed preferable to adhere to the term " albumen " in its wider application.

metabolism in the narrower sense. In that which appears as an iron-content when the red corpuscles are examined, there lies inherent the healing property of the blood. Accordingly, iron also appears in the gastric juice, and as iron-oxide in the chyle. In all of these, sources are created for counterbalancing processes as against the processes of the nerves.

Iron appears, upon examination of the blood, in such a way as to represent the only metal which, within the human organism, has a tendency towards the power of crystallization. It thus makes felt within the body forces which are in reality the outer, physical, mineral forces of Nature. These forces are present within the human organism as a force-system whose whole orientation is in the sense of outer, physical Nature; but it is perpetually being overcome by the Ego-organization.

We have, therefore, two systems of forces: the one has its origin in the nerve-processes, the other in the blood-formation. In the nerves, processes of disease unfold, but only go so far that the perpetual counter-influence of the blood-processes is still able to heal them. These nerve-processes are brought about in the nervous substance—and hence in the organism as a whole—by the astral body. The blood-processes, on the other hand, are those in which the Ego-organization within the human body confronts outer physical Nature, which is here continued into the body and subjugated by the Ego-organization to its own formative process.

In this inter-relationship we can directly apprehend the essential processes of sickening and healing. If there arise within the organism intensifications of those activities which are present in their normal measure in all that is stimulated by the nervous process, illness ensues. And if we can confront such processes by others, representing intensifications of certain influences of external Nature within the body, a healing effect will be brought about if these workings of outer Nature are mastered by the organism of the Ego and are such as to counterbalance the opposing morbid process.

Milk contains but small quantities of iron. Milk, indeed, is the substance which represents, in its activities as such, the very smallest measure of the sickening forces. The blood, on the other hand, must perpetually expose itself to all the influences of disease; it requires therefore the organized iron, that is to say the iron which has been received into the organization of the Ego—the hæmatin—as a constant remedy or means of healing.

For a remedy which is intended to influence a morbid condition appearing in the inner organization (or one that is brought about externally but takes its course within the organism), the first point is to discover how and to what extent the astral organization is working so as to bring about, at some point in the body, a disintegration of albumen such as is normally called into play by the nervous organization. Let us assume that we have to do with stoppages or congestions in the abdominal region. We can observe, in the acute attacks of pain, an excessive activity of the astral body. In such a case the above-described event has taken place in the intestinal system.

The question now is: How is the intensified astral influence to be counterbalanced? This is done by introducing into the blood substances which can be taken hold of by just that part of the Ego-organization which works in the intestinal system. Such substances are potassium and sodium. If we introduce them into the body in some suitable preparation—or through the organization of a plant such as *anagallis arvensis*—we relieve the astral body of its excessive nervous influence. We bring about a transition of the excessive action of the astral body, to the influences—taken hold of by the Ego-organization—of the above-named substances out of the blood.

56

If the substance is given in mineral form, we shall have to take care that the potassium or sodium enter the circulation of the blood in the right way, so as to arrest the metamorphosis of albumen before the point of disintegration. This may be done by the use of auxiliary remedies, or better still by combining the potassium or sodium in the preparation with sulphur. Sulphur has the peculiar property of helping to arrest the disintegration of albumen. It holds the organizing forces of albuminous substance, as it were, together. Brought into the circulation in such a way as to maintain its union with the potassium or sodium, it will make this influence felt in the region of those organs to which potassium or sodium has a special affinity. This applies, in fact, to the intestinal organs.

CHAPTER VIII

ACTIVITIES WITHIN THE HUMAN ORGANISM

Diabetes Mellitus

THROUGH all its members, the activities which the human body unfolds must have their source and impulse in the organism itself and there alone. Whatsoever is received from outside, must either merely provide the occasion for the organism to unfold its own activities, or the foreign activity it introduces must be no longer distinguishable from the internal action of the body once it has entered into the latter.

The essential nourishment of man contains, for instance, carbohydrates. Among these are the substances of the character of starch, which unfold their activity in the plant organism. They come into the human body in the condition they have been able to reach in the plant. Now in this condition starch is a foreign body. The human organism evolves no activity in the direction of any activities that starch, in the state in which it first enters the body, is able to develop. The starch-like substance produced, for example, in the human liver (namely, glycogen) is something altogether different from vegetable starch. In grape-sugar, on the other hand, we have a substance kindling activities of the same kind as those that belong to the human organism itself. Starch, therefore, cannot remain as starch in the human body. To unfold an influence that plays any real part in the body, it must first be transformed. It is in effect transformed into sugar by permeation with ptyalin in the oral cavity.

Albumens and fats are not transformed by ptyalin. To begin with they come into the stomach as foreign substances. The albumens are here transformed by the secreted pepsin, giving rise to products of disintegration down to the peptones. The peptones are substances whose impulses of action coincide already with those of the body itself. Fat, on the other hand, remains unchanged in the stomach also. It is only changed when it reaches the region of the pancreas, where it gives rise to substances that appear on examination of the dead organism as glycerine and fatty acids.

Now the transformation of starch into sugar continues through the whole process of digestion. Transformation of starch also takes place in the gastric juice if it has not already been accomplished by the ptyalin.

Where the transformation of starch is achieved by ptyalin, the process stands at the boundary of that which takes place, in man, in the domain referred to in the second chapter as the organization of the Ego. It is in this domain that the first transformation of materials, received into the human body from the outer world, takes place. Grape-sugar is a substance that can work in the sphere of the Ego-organization. Corresponding to it is the taste of sweetness, which also has its being in the Ego-organization.

If sugar is produced from starch in the gastric juice, it shows that the Ego-organization penetrates into the region of the digestive system. For conscious experience, the sensation of sweet taste is absent in this case. Nevertheless, the same thing that goes on in consciousness—in the domain of the Ego-organization—while the sensation " sweet " is experienced, has now penetrated into the unconscious regions of the human body, where the Ego-organization thus becomes active.

Now, in the regions of which we are unconscious, the astral body—in the sense that was explained in Chapter II—comes into play. The astral body is active when starch is transformed into sugar in the stomach.

Man can only be conscious through those workings in his Ego-organization where the latter is in no way disturbed or overpowered by other influences, but able to unfold itself to the full. This is the case in the domain where the ptyalin influences are primarily situated. In the realm of the pepsin influences, the astral body overwhelms the Ego-organization. The Ego-activity becomes submerged in the astral. Thus, in the sphere of material substance, we can trace the Ego-organization by the presence of sugar. Where sugar is, there is the Ego-organization; where sugar comes into being, there the Ego-organization emerges, humanizing the sub-human (vegetative and animal) bodily activities.

Now sugar occurs as a product of excretion in *Diabetes mellitus.* Here the Ego-organization appears in the human body in such a form as to work destructively. If we observe it in any other region of its activity, we find that the Ego-organization dives down into the astral. Sugar, consumed as such, is in the Ego-organization, where it acts as a stimulus giving rise to the taste of sweetness. Starch, consumed and transformed into sugar by ptyalin or in the gastric juice, reveals the action—in the oral cavity or in the stomach, as the case may be—of the astral body, which is working with the Ego-organization and submerging the latter.

Now sugar is present in the blood as well. The

blood, as it circulates with its sugar-content, carries the Ego-organization through and through the body. But in this case the Ego-organization is everywhere held in equilibrium by the working of the human organization as a whole. We saw in Chapter II how the human being contains, besides the Ego-organization and astral body, the etheric body and the physical. These too receive the Ego-organization into themselves and contain it. So long as this is the case, sugar is not secreted in the urine. The condition of the Ego-organization, as it carries the sugar through the body, is revealed in those bodily processes which are essentially bound up with sugar.

In a healthy man sugar can only appear in the urine if consumed too copiously as sugar, or again, if alcohol is consumed in excess. Alcohol enters directly into the processes of the body without intermediate products of transformation. In both these cases the sugar-process appears independently as such, alongside of the other activities in the human being.

In *Diabetes mellitus* the case is as follows: The Ego-organization, as it dives down into the astral and etheric realm, is so weakened that it can no longer effectively accomplish its action upon the sugar-substance. The sugar then undergoes in the astral and etheric realms the processes which should properly be subject to the organization of the Ego.

Diabetes is aggravated by everything that draws the Ego-organization away and impairs its effective penetration into the bodily activities. This would apply for instance to excitements occurring not singly but repeatedly, to intellectual over-exertions; or to hereditary predispositions hindering the normal co-ordination of the Ego-organization with the body as a whole.

At the same time and in connection with these things, activities take place in the head-system which ought properly to be parallel processes accompanying the operations of the soul and Spirit. They fall out of their true parallelism because the latter activities are taking place either too slowly or too quickly. It is as though the nervous system were thinking independently alongside of the thinking human being. Now this is an activity which the nervous system should only carry out during sleep. In the diabetic subject a kind of sleep is going on in the depths of the body alongside of the waking state. Hence in the further course of the disease a morbid degeneration of nervous substance takes place. It is a consequence of the deficient penetration of the organizing activity of the Ego.

The formation of boils is another collateral

symptom in Diabetes. Boils arise through an excessive activity in the domain of the etheric. The Ego-organization fails where it should properly be working. The astral activity too cannot unfold itself, for at such a point especially, it is powerless unless working in harmony with the Ego-organization. The result is an excess of etheric activity revealing itself in the formation of boils.

From all this we see that a real healing process for *Diabetes mellitus* can only be initiated if one is in a position to strengthen the Ego-organization of the patient.

CHAPTER IX

ALBUMEN IN THE HUMAN BODY

Albuminuria

OF all kinds of substance in the living body, albumen lends itself to the most manifold transformations by the formative forces of the organism. The outcome of the albuminous substance thus transformed is apparent in the forms of the organs and of the living organism as a whole. To be made use of in such a way, albumen must have the inherent faculty to resign all form that might proceed from the nature of its material constituents the moment it is summoned to subject itself within the organism to a form which the latter demands.

We thus perceive that in albumen the forces proceeding from the natures and mutual relationships of Hydrogen, Oxygen, Nitrogen, and Carbon fall asunder and disintegrate. The inorganic bindings of substance cease to take effect, and in the disintegrating albumen, organic formative forces begin to work.

Now these formative forces are bound up with the etheric body. Albumen is ever on the alert, either to be received into the action of the etheric body or to fall out of it. Removed from the living organism to which it once belonged, it assumes the tendency to become a compound, subject to the inorganic forces of hydrogen, oxygen, nitrogen, and carbon. Albumen that remains a constituent of the living body rids itself of this tendency and becomes subject to the formative forces of the etheric.

Man consumes albumen as a constituent of the food he takes. The pepsin of the stomach transforms the albumen, which is thus received from outside, as far as to the peptones. These, to begin with, are soluble albuminous substances. The transformation is then continued by the pancreatic juice.

The albumen absorbed as a constituent of food is, to begin with, a foreign body in the human organism. It still contains residual activities from the etheric processes of the living being whence it was derived. All this must be entirely removed from it, for it now has to be received into the etheric activity of the human organism.

Hence, in the course of the human process of digestion, we have to do with two kinds of albuminous substance. At the beginning of the digestive process the albumen is foreign to the human organism; at the end it is its property. Between these two conditions there is an intermediate one, where the albumen received as food has not yet entirely discarded its previous etheric actions nor yet entirely assumed the new. At this stage it is wellnigh completely inorganic. It is then subject to the influences of the human physical body alone. The physical body of man—in its form a product of the Ego-organization—contains inorganic forces and activities. It thus has a killing effect on anything that is alive. Everything that enters the realm of the Ego-organization begins to die. Hence in the physical body the Ego-organization incorporates purely inorganic substances. The action of these, though in the physical organism of man they work not in the same way as in the external lifeless world of Nature, is nevertheless inorganic: it kills what is alive. This killing action upon the living albumen takes place in that part of the digestive tract where trypsin— a constituent of the pancreatic juice—unfolds its activity.

That inorganic forces are concerned in the action of trypsin, may be gathered also from the fact that it unfolds its activity in the presence and with the help of alkali.

Until it meets the trypsin in the pancreatic fluid,

the albuminous nourishment continues to live in a manner foreign to the human organism, namely, according to the organism from which it is derived. Meeting the trypsin, it becomes lifeless. But it is only for a moment, as it were, that the albumen is lifeless in the human organism. Then it is received into the physical body in accordance with the organization of the Ego. The latter must have the force to carry over what the albumen has now become into the domain of the human etheric body. In this way the albumen constituents of food become formative material for the human organism. The foreign etheric influences, pertaining to them originally, leave the human being.

For the healthy digestion of albuminous food, man must possess a sufficiently strong Ego-organization to enable all the albumen, which the human organism needs, to pass into the domain of the human etheric body. If this is not the case, the result is an excessive activity of the etheric body. The quantity of albumen prepared by the Ego-organization, which the etheric body receives, is insufficient for its activity. The activity, intended to call to life the albumen which should be received from the Ego-organization, will then take hold of albumen that still contains the foreign etheric influences. The human being receives in his own etheric body a multitude of influences that do not

68

properly belong to it. These must now be excreted in an abnormal manner. A morbid process of excretion is the result.

This morbid excretion appears in *albuminuria*. The albumen which should be received into the domain of the etheric body is excreted. It is albumen, which, owing to the weakness of the Ego-organization, has not been able to assume the intermediate stage of the wellnigh lifeless.

Now the forces in man which bring about excretion are bound up with the domain of the astral body. In albuminuria, the astral body being forced to carry out an activity for which it is not properly adapted, its activity becomes atrophied in the regions of the body where it ought properly to unfold, namely, in the renal epithelia. The degeneration of the epithelia in the kidneys is a symptom, showing that the activity of the astral body which is intended for these organs has been diverted.

It is clear from all this where the healing process for albuminuria must enter in. The power of the Ego-organization in the pancreas, being too weak, needs to be strengthened.

CHAPTER X

FAT IN THE HUMAN ORGANISM

Deceptive Local Complexes of Symptoms

OF all substances in the organism, it is Fat that shows itself least of all as a foreign body when taken in from the outer world. More readily than any other substance, it passes over from the quality it brings with it when taken as a food to the mode of action of the human organism itself. The 80 per cent. of fat contained, for instance, in butter, passes unchanged through the domains of ptyalin and pepsin and is only transformed by the pancreatic juice—into glycerine and fatty acids. This behaviour of fat is dependent on its property of carrying with it as little as possible of the nature of a foreign organism (namely of its etheric forces and the like) into the human organism. The latter can easily incorporate it into its own activity.

This again is due to the fact that fat plays its peculiar part above all in the production of the inner warmth. Now the inner warmth is the element of the physical organism in which the

Ego-organization paramountly lives. Whatever substance is present in the human body, for the Ego-organization only so much of it comes into play as represents the evolution of warmth which its activity involves. The whole behaviour of fat shows it to be a substance which merely fills the body, is merely carried by the body, and is important for the active organization through those processes alone in which it engenders warmth. Fat that is received, for instance, as nourishment from an animal organism, takes nothing over from the animal organism into the human, except its inherent faculty to evolve heat or warmth.

Now this evolution of warmth is one of the latest processes of the metabolism. The fat received as food is therefore preserved as such throughout the first and middle processes of metabolism; its absorption only takes place in the region of the inmost activities of the body, beginning with the pancreatic fluid.

The occurrence of fat in human milk points to an exceedingly significant activity of the organism. The body does not consume this fat, but allows it to pass over into a product of secretion. Now, into this secreted fat the Ego-organization also passes over. It is on this that the form-giving, constructive power of the mother's milk depends. The mother thereby transmits her own formative forces of the Ego-organization to the child, and thus adds something more to the configurating forces which she has already transmitted by heredity.

It is a healthy mode of action when the human form-giving forces consume in the development of warmth the supply of fat that is present in the organism. On the other hand it is unhealthy if the fat is not used up by the Ego-organization with its processes of warmth, but carried over, unused, into the organism. Such fat will then give rise at one point or another in the body to an excessive power of producing warmth. The warmth thus engendered will take hold of the organism at one point or another, interfering with the remaining processes of life. It is not embraced by the Ego-organization. There arise, as it were, parasitic centres of warmth, tending to inflammatory conditions. The origin of these lies in the fact that the body develops a tendency to accumulate more fat than the Ego-organization requires for its life in inner warmth.

In the healthy organism, the animal (astral) forces will produce or receive as much fat as the Ego-organization is able to translate into warmth-processes and, in addition, as much as is required to keep the mechanism of muscle and bone in order. The warmth that the body needs will then

72

be engendered. If the animal forces supply the Ego-organization with an insufficient quantity of fat, it will be starved for warmth and thus obliged to withdraw the warmth it needs from the activities of the organs. The latter then become inwardly stiff and brittle. Their essential processes take place too sluggishly. We then witness the appearance, at one point or another, of morbid processes, for an understanding of which it will be necessary to recognize if and how they are due to a general deficiency of fat.

If, as in the case already mentioned, there is an excess of fat, giving rise to parasitic centres of warmth, organs will be seized in such a way as to become active beyond their normal measure. Tendencies will arise towards an excessive absorption of food, so as to overload the organism. It need not imply that the person becomes an excessive eater. It may be, for instance, that the metabolic activity of the organism supplies too much substance to a certain organ of the head, withdrawing it from organs of the lower body and from the secretory processes. The action of the organs thus deprived will then be lowered in vitality. The secretions of the glands, for instance, may become deficient. The liquid constituents of the body are brought into an unhealthy state with respect to their relative proportions of admixture.

For instance, the secretion of bile may become too great compared with that of pancreatic fluid. Once again, it will be important to recognize how a complex of symptoms arising locally is truly to be estimated, inasmuch as it may proceed in one way or another from an unhealthy activity of fat.

CHAPTER XI

CONFIGURATION OF THE HUMAN BODY

Gout

ABSORPTION of albumen is a process related to the one side of the inner operations in the human organism, namely to that which arises on the basis of the absorption of substances. Every operation of this kind eventuates in growth, creation of form, or re-creation of substantial content. All that is related to the unconscious functions of the organism, belongs to this domain.

The processes of this kind are, however, confronted by others, which represent excretions. (These may be excretions in the proper sense — excretions passing outward; but they may also be processes of " secretion " where the product is further elaborated internally, in the forming and substantiating of the body.) These are the processes which provide the material foundation of conscious experience. Through processes of the former kind the force of consciousness is lowered, whenever they exceed the measure which this latter kind can hold in equilibrium.

A most remarkable excretory process is that of uric acid. The astral body is active in this excretion, which has to take place throughout the organism. In the urine it takes place to a high degree; but in a very finely divided way it is also going on, for example, in the brain. In the secretion of uric acid in the urine the astral body is paramountly active, while the part played by the Ego-organization is only subsidiary. In the secretion of uric acid in the brain, on the other hand, the Ego-organization is the important factor and the astral body falls into the background.

Now in the whole organism it is the astral body that mediates between the activity of the Ego-organization, and the etheric and physical bodies. The Ego-organization must carry lifeless substances and forces into the organs. Only through this impregnation of the organs with inorganic material can man become the conscious being that he is. Organic substances, organic forces, would lower human consciousness to the dim level of the animal.

The action of the astral body inclines the organs to receive the inorganic impregnations of the Ego-system. Its function is in fact to prepare the way for the organization of the Ego.

We see, therefore, that in the lower parts of the human organism the activity of the astral body has the upper hand. Here the uric acid substances must not be received into the organism; they must be excreted copiously, and under the influence of this excretion the impregnation with inorganic material must be prevented. The more uric acid is excreted, the more copious is the activity of the astral body, while that of the Ego-organization impregnating the body with inorganic materials is correspondingly decreased.

In the brain, on the other hand, the activity of the astral body is far less. Very little uric acid is secreted, while all the more inorganic material is deposited through the agency of the Ego-system.

The Ego-organization cannot master large quantities of uric acid, and they thus fall under the action of the astral body. Small quantities, on the other hand, enter the organization of the Ego, and there provide the foundation for the forming of inorganic elements under the direction of the latter.

In the healthy organism there must be a right economy in the distribution of uric acid through the several regions. Whatever belongs to the system of nerves and senses must be provided with as much uric acid as the Ego-organization can make use of, and no more; while, for the system of metabolism and the limbs, the Ego-activity must be suppressed and the astral enabled to unfold its action in the more copious secretion of uric acid.

Now since it is the astral body that makes way for the Ego-activities in the organs, a true distribution in the depositing of uric acid must be regarded as an essential factor in human health. For in this, the right relation between the Ego-organization and the astral body in any organ or system of organs will find expression.

Let us assume that in some organ, in which the Ego-organization should predominate over the astral activity, the latter begins to gain the upper hand. This can only apply to an organ where the excretion of uric acid beyond a certain measure is impossible by virtue of its structural arrangement. The organ becomes overloaded with uric acid which is uncontrolled by the Ego-organization. The astral body begins to bring about a secretion of uric acid nevertheless, and since the organs of exit are lacking in such a region, the uric acid is deposited not outwardly but in the organism. And if it finds its way to places in the body where the Ego-organization is unable to take a sufficiently active part, we shall there have to do with inorganic material—*i.e.*, with something which is proper to the Ego-organization only, but which the latter resigns to the action of the astral. Morbid centres arise, where sub-human (animal) processes insert themselves into the human organism.

This is the case in gout. If gout is reputed frequently to develop as a result of inherited tendencies, it is due to the simple fact that when the forces of inheritance predominate, the astral-animal nature becomes especially active and the Ego-organization is thereby repressed.

We shall, however, penetrate the matter more clearly if we look for the true cause of gout in this: Substances are introduced into the human body in the process of nourishment, which the activity of the organism is not strong enough to divest of their foreign nature. The Ego-organization, being weak, is unable to lead them over into the etheric body, and they thus remain in the region of astral activities. If an articular cartilage or a portion of connective tissue become overcharged with uric acid and, as a result, over-burdened with inorganic materials and forces, it shows that in these parts of the body the Ego's activity is supplanted by the operation of the astral. And since the whole form of the human organism is an outcome of the organization of the Ego, this abnormality must necessarily give rise to a deformation of the organs. In effect, the human organism will then strive away from its true and proper form.

CHAPTER XII

CONSTRUCTIVE AND EXCRETIVE PROCESSES IN THE HUMAN ORGANISM

LIKE other living organisms, the human body is formed out of the semi-fluid state. In the process of its formation, a perpetual supply of aeriform materials is however necessary. The most important of these is the Oxygen transmitted by the breath.

We may consider in the first place a solid constituent of the body—the structure of the bony system, for example. It is separated out from a semi-liquid material. In this process, the Ego-organization is active, as anyone may observe by tracing the actual course of development of the bony system. For, in the embryonic period and in childhood, the bony system develops in the same measure in which the human being receives his human form and figure, the characteristic expression of the Ego-nature. The transformation of albumen which underlies this process first eliminates the (astral and etheric) foreign forces from the albumin-

80

ous substance. The albumen then passes through the inorganic state, and in so doing, it has to become fluid. In this condition, the Ego-organization, working in the element of warmth, takes hold of it and brings it into the sphere of the etheric body of the man himself. It thus becomes human albumen, but it still has a long way to go before the transformation into bony substance is achieved.

After its transformation into human albumen, it must first be prepared for the processes of receiving and transforming the calcium carbonate, calcium phosphate, and the like. To this end it must undergo an intermediate stage. It must be subjected to the influences that accompany the absorption of aeriform substance, which carries the transformation-products of the carbohydrates into the albumen. The substances which thus arise can provide a basis for the formations of the several organs. They represent, not the finished substances of the organs—liver-substance or bone-substance for example—but a more general, less differentiated substance from out of which the several organs of the body are then built up. The Ego-organization is active in moulding the final shapes of the organs. In the organic substance, as yet undifferentiated, to which we here refer, the astral body is at work. In the animal, the astral body also takes upon itself the task of moulding the final forms of the organs; in man, the activity of the astral body and, with it, the animal nature as such, persists only as a general underlying foundation for the organization of the Ego. In man the animal creation is not carried to a conclusion; it is interrupted half-way and the Ego-organization then comes in to crown it, as it were, with the creation of the human.

Now, the Ego-organization lives entirely in states of warmth. It derives the several organs from the undifferentiated astral nature. It works upon the undifferentiated substance with which the astral nature provides it, by enhancing or lowering the states of warmth of the nascent organs.

If the Ego-organization lowers the state of warmth, inorganic materials enter the substance and a hardening process sets in. The basis is thus provided for the creation of the bones. Salt-like substances are absorbed.

If, on the other hand, the Ego-organization enhances the state of warmth, organs are produced, whose characteristic action is to dissolve the organic substance, leading it over into a liquid or aeriform condition.

Assume now, the Ego-organization finds that not enough warmth is being developed in the organism to enable the states of warmth to be sufficiently enhanced for those organs for which such enhancement is necessary. Organs whose proper functioning lies in the direction of a dissolving process will then fall into a hardening activity. They assume in a morbid way the same tendency which, in the bones, is healthy.

Now the bone, once it has been formed, is an organ which the Ego-organization releases from its domain. It then enters a condition where it is no longer taken hold of by the Ego-organization inwardly, but only in an outward way. Removed thenceforth from the domain of growing and organizing processes, it serves the Ego in a merely mechanical capacity, to carry out the movements of the body. Only a relic of the inner organizing activity of the Ego continues to permeate it, and this must go on throughout the human being's life, for the bony system must, after all, remain as an integral organic part within the body; it must not be allowed to fall entirely out of the sphere of life.

The blood vessels are the organs which, for the reason above mentioned, may pass into a formative activity similar to that of the bones. We then have the calcifying disease of the arteries known as Sclerosis. In this disease the Ego-organization is, in a certain sense, driven out of these systems of organs.

The opposite is the case when the Ego-organization fails to find the adequate lowering of the state of warmth which is needed for the region of the bones. The bones then assume a condition similar to those organs which normally unfold a dissolving kind of activity. Owing to the deficient hardening process, they are no longer able to provide a basis for the incorporation of salts. Thus the final process in the development of the bone-formations, which properly belongs to the organizing domain of the Ego, fails to take place. The astral activity is not arrested at the proper point. Tendencies of deformation are the necessary outcome; for the healthy creation of the human form and figure is only possible within the realm of the Ego-organization. We here have the diseases of the character of Rickets.

From all this it becomes evident how the human organs are connected with their several activities. The bone comes into being in the realm of the Ego-organization, and it still continues to serve the same when its formation is concluded—when the Ego-organization no longer forms and creates it, but uses it freely in executing the voluntary movements. So it is, in like manner, with that which arises in the astral realm of organization. In the astral domain, undifferentiated substances and forces are created. These substances and forces occur throughout the body as an underlying basis for the differentiated organ-forming processes. The astral activity carries these processes up to a certain stage and then makes use of them. The whole human organism is permeated by semi-liquid material, in which an astrally directed activity holds sway.

The astral activity finds expression in the secretions which are made use of to form the organism in the direction of its higher members. Secretions with this directive tendency are to be seen in the products of the glands which play so important a part in the economy of the organism and its functions. In addition to these inward secretions, we then have the processes that are excretions in the proper sense, towards the outer world. But we make a mistake if we regard the excretions merely as those portions of the food consumed which the organism cannot make use of and therefore discards. For the important thing is not the mere fact that the organism throws certain substances out, but rather, that it goes through the activities which result in the excretions. The exercise of these activities is something that the organism needs for its subsistence. This kind of activity is no less necessary than that by which the substances are received into the organism, or secreted and deposited internally. In the healthy relationship of these two kinds of activities, there lies the very essence of organic life and action.

Thus, in the outward excretions we see the result of an activity astrally directed. And if the excreta contain substances which have been carried to the inorganic nature, then the Ego-organization, too, is living in them. Indeed, this part of the Ego-organization's life is of peculiar importance. For the force that is applied to excretions of this kind creates, as it were, an inward counter-pressure or reaction. And this latter is a necessary factor for the healthy existence of the organism. Thus the uric acid, which is separated outward in the urine, creates as an inward reaction the proper tendency of the body as a whole to sleep. Too little uric acid in the urine and too much in the blood will give rise to a period of sleep insufficient for the healthy life of the organism.

CHAPTER XIII

ON THE NATURE OF ILLNESS AND HEALING

PAIN, wheresoever in the organism it occurs, is a conscious experience in the astral body and the Ego. Both of these—the astral body and the Ego, each in its own way—are intimately connected with the etheric and physical body so long as man is in the waking state. When sleep takes place, the physical and etheric body perform the organic actions alone, the astral body and Ego being separated from them.

In sleep the organism returns to the modes of action which belong to the starting point of its development, namely, to the embryo period and early childhood. In waking life the processes predominate which take place at its conclusion—in old age and death.

At the starting point of man's development the activity of the etheric body predominates over that of the astral. Then, gradually in the course of life, the activity of the astral grows more intense while that of the etheric body declines. Nor does the etheric body regain, even in sleep, the intensity it had at the beginning of man's life. It preserves the degree of intensity which, in relation to the astral, it has developed in the course of life.

In every age of life, to every organ of the human body a certain intensity of etheric activity is properly assigned and corresponds moreover to a certain intensity of the astral. On the presence of these true relationships it depends, whether or no the astral body can properly adapt itself and enter into the etheric. If through a lowering of etheric vitality it is unable to do so, pain ensues. If on the other hand the etheric body becomes active beyond its normal measure, the penetration of astral and etheric workings grows unusually intense. This expresses itself in a sense of pleasure, comfort and delight. We must however bear in mind that pleasure enhanced beyond a certain point passes over into pain, likewise pain into pleasure. If this were not borne in mind what is here said might seem in contradiction with some former explanations.

An organ becomes ill when the etheric activity which is properly its due cannot unfold. Take, for instance, that metabolic action which is continued, from the digestive process, into the organism as a whole. If the products of the metabolism are everywhere transmitted without residue into the

88

activity and substantial formation of the body, it is a sign that the etheric body is working rightly. If on the other hand substances are deposited along the paths of metabolism without entering into the general action of the organism, it shows that the activity of the etheric is lowered. The physical processes normally stimulated by the astral body— processes which only serve the organism when confined to their own sphere—exceed their proper limits and infringe on the sphere of the etheric. Processes arise whose existence is due to the pre-dominance of the astral body. They are processes which have their proper place where the ageing and disintegrating of the body sets in.

The point now is to bring about a proper harmony between the etheric activity and the astral. The etheric body must be strengthened, the astral weakened. This can be done by bringing the physical substances, which the etheric body has to assimilate, into a condition where they lend themselves more readily to its influence than they do in the disease. Likewise the Ego-organization must be supplied with added strength; for the astral body, with the animal orientation of its activity, is held more in check when the Ego-system is strengthened in the direction of its human organizing power.

The way to penetrate these matters with clear

knowledge will be found when we observe the kind of effects which a particular substance unfolds on the paths of metabolism. Take sulphur for instance. It is contained in albumen. It is indeed fundamental to the whole process which takes place in the absorption of albuminous food. From the foreign etheric nature, it passes through the inorganic state into the etheric action of the human organism itself. It is found in the fibrous tissues of the organs, in the brain, in the nails and hair. Thus it finds its way along the paths of metabolism even to the periphery of the organism. In all these ways, sulphur proves to be a substance which plays an essential part in the reception of albumens into the domain of the human etheric body.

Now the question arises, does sulphur also play a part in the transition from the domain of etheric action to that of astral, and has it anything to do with the Ego-organization? It does not combine appreciably with inorganic substances introduced into the body, so as to form salts or acids. Such a combination would provide the basis for a reception of the sulphur processes into the astral body and Ego-organization. We see, therefore, that sulphur does not penetrate into these regions. It unfolds its activity in the realm of the physical body and the etheric. This is also shown by the fact that an increased supply of sulphur to the organism gives rise to feelings of giddiness, lowerings of consciousness. Sleep, too—*i.e.* the condition of the body when the astral and Ego-organization are psychologically inactive—grows more intense when the supply of sulphur is increased.

From all this we can see that sulphur, introduced as a medicament, will make the physical activities of the organism more inclined to submit to the active influence of the etheric than they are in the condition of disease.

With phosphorus the case is different. It is present in the human organism as phosphoric acid and phosphoric salts, in albumens, in the fibrous tissues, in the brain, and in the bones. It tends towards the inorganic substances which have their significance in the domain of the Ego-organization. It stimulates the conscious activity of man. Thus it also conditions sleep—though by an opposite process, namely by previous stimulation of the conscious activity; while sulphur favours sleep, as we have seen, by enhancing the unconscious activities of the physical and etheric. Phosphorous is present as calcium phosphate in the bones, *i.e.* in those organs which are subject to the Ego-organization, not where it works from within in processes of growth, regulation of metabolism, and the like, but where it uses the outer mechanism of the system for the movements of the body.

As a remedy, therefore, phosphorus will be effective when the morbid condition is a hypertrophy of the astral domain over the Ego-organization and the latter needs to be strengthened in order to repress the astral.

Consider the case of rickets. It was explained before, how rickets consists in a hypertrophy of etheric-astral activity and leads to a defective action of the Ego-organization. If this disease is treated first with sulphur in the proper way, the etheric activity is strengthened in relation to the astral; and if after this has been done, a phosphorus treatment is made to follow, the healing effect which has been prepared in the etheric organization is led over to that of the " Ego," and the disease is met from two different sides. (We are aware that the efficacy of the phosphorus treatment of rickets is disputed; but none of the cures hitherto attempted represent the method which is here described.)

CHAPTER XIV

THERAPEUTIC METHOD OF THOUGHT

SILICA (silicic acid) carries its influences along the paths of metabolism into those parts of the human organism where the living becomes lifeless. It occurs in the blood, through which the forces of configuration have to take their course. It occurs also in the hair, *i.e.*, where the forming and shaping process finds its outward culmination; and we find it in the bones, where the process of formation culminates inwardly. It appears in the urine as a product of excretion.

It constitutes the physical basis of the Ego-organization. For the latter has a forming and configurating action. The Ego-organization needs the silica—it needs it right into the frontier regions of the organism where its form-giving action meets with the outer and the inner (unconscious) world. At the periphery of the organism where the hair contains silica, the human organization meets with the unconscious outer world. In the bones it meets the unconscious inner world, in which the Will is working.

In the healthy human organism the physical foundation of consciousness must unfold between these two fields of action of silica. The silica has a twofold function. Within, it sets a limit to the mere processes of growth, nourishment, etc. Outwardly, it shuts off the activities of external Nature from the interior of the body, so that the organism within its own domain is not obliged to continue the mere workings of external Nature, but enabled to unfold its own activities.

In its early stages of existence the human organism is most highly equipped with silicic acid in those localities where tissues with strong formative forces are situated. Thence the silica unfolds its activity towards the two limiting regions, creating between them the space in which the organs of conscious life can arise. In the healthy human organism, these are primarily the sense-organs. We must, however, bear in mind that the sensory life permeates the whole organism. The mutual interaction of the organs depends upon the fact that the one organ is continually perceiving the influences of the other. In organs which are not sense-organs in the proper meaning of the term— for instance in the liver, spleen, or kidneys—the perception is so slight as to remain in normal waking life beneath the threshold of consciousness. Nevertheless, every organ—besides serving this or that function within the body—is in addition a sense-organ.

The whole human organism is in fact permeated with perceptions which influence one another mutually; and it must be so if all the different processes are to work in it together healthily.

Now all this is dependent on a right distribution of the activities of silica. We can even go so far as to speak of a silica-organism, permeating the organism as a whole. This " silica organism " conditions the mutual sensitiveness of the organs on which the healthy life and activity depend. It determines their right inward and outward relationships: inwardly their relation to the unfolding of the life of soul and Spirit; and outwardly, in the sense that it provides in each case for the proper exclusion of the activities of external Nature.

This special organism of silica will only be working rightly, if silica is present in the body in such quantities that the organization of the Ego is able to make full use of it. Any remaining amounts of silica, the astral organization which lies beneath that of the Ego must have the power to excrete —either through the urine or in some other way.

Excessive quantities of silica, which are neither excreted nor taken hold of by the Ego-organization, will be deposited as foreign substances in the body. Through the very form-creating tendency whereby—in the right quantity—they serve the Ego-organization, they will then disturb it. Excessive quantities of silica, introduced into the organism, will thus impair the workings of the stomach and intestinal system, giving rise to conditions of indigestion. For it will be the task of the digestive tract to get rid of the excessive form-creating tendency. Where the fluid element should predominate, desiccation will be brought about. This is most plainly evident when the excessive introduction of silica is followed by psychological disturbances of equilibrium, behind which the corresponding organic effects are unmistakable. One feels a sense of giddiness and is unable to repress the tendency to fall asleep; one feels unable to direct the perceptions of sight and hearing in the proper way. Nay, one may even have a feeling as though the impressions of the senses became congested and held up at the point where they should be continued into the interior of the nervous system. All this shows how silica presses out towards the periphery of the body; and how, if it arrives there in excessive quantities, it disturbs the normal configurating process by introducing a foreign influence of configuration. Towards the inner boundary of the form-creating process too, disturbances occur. One feels a difficulty in directing the movements of the body, and experiences pain in the joints. All these conditions may eventuate in processes of inflammation, arising wherever the foreign force of configuration, introduced by the silica, makes itself felt too strongly.

Now this points at the same time to the healing forces which silica can unfold in the human organism. Assume that an organ—not a sense-organ in the proper meaning of the term—becomes over-sensitive in its unconscious power of perception with respect to the parts of the organism external to it. We shall then observe a disturbance in the functions of this organ. We shall be able to deal effectively with the morbid condition if we are in a position to eliminate the over-sensitiveness by administering silica. It will, however, be necessary so to influence the organic workings of the body that the added silica takes effect in the neighbourhood of the diseased organ, and does not work upon the whole body with a general influence of the kind above described.

By a combination of silica with other remedies the desired result can be brought about. The silica introduced into the organism will then find its way to the organ where it is needed, whence— if properly administered—it will be carried out again as a product of excretion without doing harm to other organs of the system.

In another case the sensitiveness of an organ to the activities of the remaining organs may be unduly lowered. We then have to do with an accumulation of the silica-activity in the neighbourhood of this organ. It will be necessary, therefore, to find a means of influencing the silica-activity of the whole organism, so as to deprive the localized action of its excessive power. Or again, the removal of the silica may be stimulated by the use of laxatives. The former method is to be preferred, for an accumulation of silica in one locality generally calls forth a corresponding deficiency in another. The distribution of the localized silica-activity over the whole organism may be brought about, for instance, by a sulphur cure. The reader will perceive why this is so, if he will refer again to another chapter where the influences of sulphur are characterized.

CHAPTER XV

THE METHOD OF HEALING

OUR knowledge of remedial effects depends upon our clear perception of the forces that unfold in the world external to man. For in order to bring about a healing process, we must bring into the organism substances which will distribute themselves in it in such a way that the morbid process gradually passes over into a normal one. It is of the essence of a morbid process, that something is going on within the organism which refuses to become an integral part of its activities. A morbid process has this feature in common with a process of external Nature. We may say in effect: If there arises within the organism a process similar to one of external Nature, illness ensues. Such a process may take hold of the physical organism or of the etheric. Either the astral body or the Ego will then have to fulfil a task which they do not normally fulfil. In a period of life when they should be unfolding in free activity of soul, they have to return perforce to the functions of an earlier age—in some cases even as far back as the embryonic period. They have to assist in creating physical and etheric formations which should already have passed into the domain of the physical and etheric organism. Nurtured in the earliest periods of human life by the astral body and Ego-organization, these formations are afterwards taken over by the physical and etheric organism alone. Altogether, the development of the human organism depends upon this: Originally the entire form and configuration of the physical and etheric body proceed from the activity of the astral body and Ego-organization. Then, with increasing age, the astral and Ego-activities go on of their own accord within the physical and etheric organization. If on the other hand they fail to do so, the astral body and Ego-organization will have to interpose, at a later stage of their development, in a way for which they are no longer properly adapted.

Let us assume that we have to do with abdominal congestions. The physical and etheric organizations are failing to carry out, in the corresponding parts of the human body, the activities which were transmitted to them at a former age of life. The astral and Ego-activities have to interpose, and they are thereby weakened for their other functions in the organism. They are no longer present where they ought to be: for instance, in the formation of the nerves that go into the muscles. Paralytic symptoms arise as a result, in certain parts of the organism.

It will then be necessary to bring into the body substances which can relieve the astral and Ego-organization of the activity that does not properly belong to them. We find, that the processes which work in the production of powerful essential oils in the plant organism, notably in the formation of the flower, are able to fulfil this purpose. The same applies to certain substances containing phosphorus; but we must see to it that the phosphorus is so mingled with other substances as to unfold its action in the intestinal canal and not in the metabolism that lies outside this region.

If it is a case of inflammatory conditions in the skin, here too the astral body and Ego-organization are unfolding an abnormal activity. They are then withdrawn from the influences which they ought to bring to bear on organs situated more internally. In effect, they reduce the sensitiveness of internal organs. These again, owing to their lessened sensitiveness, will cease to carry out their proper functions. In this way abnormal conditions may arise, for instance in the action of the liver; and the digestion may be badly influenced. If now we introduce silica into the body, the activities which the astral and Ego-organization have been devoting to the skin are relieved. The normal inward activity of these organizations is set free again and a healing process is thus initiated.

Again, we may be confronted by morbid conditions manifesting themselves in an abnormal heartbeat. In such a case, an abnormal action of the astral organism is influencing the circulation of the blood. The astral activity is correspondingly weakened for the processes in the brain. Epileptiform conditions arise, since the weakened astral activity in the head organism involves an undue tension and exertion of the etheric activities allotted to that region. We may then introduce into the system the gum-like substance obtainable from *levisticum* (lovage)—as a decoction, or preferably in the somewhat modified form of a special preparation. The activity of the astral body, wrongly absorbed by the circulation, is then set free, and the astral activity for the brain system correspondingly strengthened.

In all these cases the real direction of the morbid activities must be determined by a proper diagnosis. Take the last mentioned case. It may be in fact that the disturbance in the interplay of the etheric and astral bodies proceeds originally from the circulation. The brain symptoms are then a consequence and we can proceed with a cure along the lines above described.

But the opposite may also be the case. The original cause of irregularity may arise between the astral and etheric activities in the brain system. Then the irregular circulation and abnormal heart-beat will be the consequence. In such a case we shall have to introduce sulphates, for example, into the metabolic process. These work on the etheric organization of the brain in such a way as to call forth in it a strong force of attraction to the astral body. The effect can be observed in the consequent improvement in initiative of thought, in the sphere of volition, and in the patient's general state of composure and control. It will probably be necessary to supplement this treatment by the use, for instance, of a copper salt, so as to assist the astral forces in regaining their renewed influence upon the circulatory system.

We shall observe that the organism as a whole returns to its regular activity when the excessive action of the astral and Ego-organism in some part of the body, conditioned by the physical and the etheric, is replaced by an activity externally induced. The organism has an inherent tendency to balance and readjust its own deficiencies. Hence it will restore itself to a right condition if an existing irregularity is regulated artificially, for a period of time, by opposing the process internally induced, which must be made to cease, with a similar process brought about by external agencies.

CHAPTER XVI

KNOWLEDGE OF MEDICAMENTS

TO judge of the efficacy of any substances for remedial purposes, we must be able to estimate in the first place the potential forces and influences —within the human organism and without it— which they contain. In this connection the reactions which ordinary Chemistry investigates come into consideration only to a small extent. The important thing is, to observe those effects which result from the inner constitution of the forces in a substance in relation to the forces that radiate outward from the Earth and in towards it.

From this point of view we may consider grey antimony ore for an example. Antimony shows a strong relationship to the sulphur compounds of other metals. Sulphur possesses a number of properties which only remain constant within— comparatively speaking—narrow limits. It is sensitive to processes of Nature such as heating, combustion, etc. This also makes it able to play an important part in the albuminous substances which, as we have seen, have the power to free themselves entirely from earthly forces and enter the domain of etheric activity. Antimony, with its peculiar affinity to sulphur, will readily partake in this intimate connection with the etheric forces. Hence antimony is easy to introduce into the activity of albumen in the human body, and it will help the latter in its etheric action when the organism itself, through some morbid condition, is unable to transform an albuminous substance introduced from without, so as to make it an integral part of its own activity.

But antimony shows other peculiarities as well. Wherever it can do so, it tends to assume a radiant (" starry ") configuration. It distributes itself in lines which strive away from the Earth, towards the forces that are active in the Ether. With antimony, we thus introduce into the human organism something that comes to meet the influences of the etheric body half-way. That which antimony undergoes in the Seiger process also points to its etheric activity. It assumes a delicate fibrous texture. Now the Seiger process is a process which begins, as it were, physically from below, and passes upward into the etheric. Antimony enters organically into this transition.

Antimony oxidizes at a red heat. In process of combustion it gives off a white smoke, which, deposited on a cold surface, produces the " flowers of antimony."

Moreover, it has a certain force of opposition to electrical influences. Under certain conditions, when deposited electrolytically on the cathode, it will readily explode by contact with a metallic point.

All this shows that antimony has a quick tendency to pass into the etheric element the moment the requisite conditions are given even to a slight degree. To the spiritual seer these many details are merely valuable as signs and indications of the truth, for he beholds directly the relationship between the Ego's activity and the working of antimony. He sees in effect how the antimony processes, when brought into the human organism, work in the same way as the Ego-organization.

The blood as it flows through the human organism shows a tendency to coagulate. This tendency, above all, stands under the influence of the Ego-organization, by which it must be regulated properly. Blood is an intermediate organic product. The blood-substance, as it originates, has undergone processes which are already on the way to the fully human organization, i.e., to the organization of the Ego. But to enter the inner configuration of this human organism it still has further processes to undergo, the nature of which may be recognized from the following: When removed from the body, the blood coagulates. It thus shows that it has in it the tendency to coagulate, and that within the organism it must be perpetually prevented from doing so. Now the power that hinders the coagulation of the blood is the very power by which it is made an integral part of the human organism. It enters the inner configuration of the body by virtue of the form-forces which lie just on the point to coagulation. If coagulation actually took place, life would be endangered.

Hence if we are dealing with a morbid condition where the body is deficient in these forces directed to the coagulation of the blood, antimony in one form or another will have a remedial effect.

The configurating process of the body is in all essentials a transformation of albuminous substance, whereby the latter comes into connection with mineralizing forces. Such forces are contained for instance in calcium. We have a graphic illustration of the facts in the formation of the oyster shell. The oyster must rid itself of the elements which are present in the shell, in order to preserve the albuminous substance in its own inherent nature. A similar thing happens in the shell-formation of the egg.

In the oyster the calcium nature is secreted and

separated out, in order not to be incorporated in the albumen activities. In the human organism the opposite is the case; the calcium element must be incorporated. The action of the albumen alone must be transmuted into a mode of action wherein an essential part is played by the inner form-giving forces, which the Ego-organization is able to evoke in the element of calcium. This has to take place in the formation of the blood. Now antimony counteracts the calcium-excreting force. Where the albumen tends to preserve its own form, antimony, by virtue of its relationship to the etheric element, leads it over into the formless condition where it is receptive to the influence of calcium and similar agencies.

Take the case of typhoid fever. The morbid condition clearly consists in a deficient transmutation of albuminous substance, into blood-substance with its power of configuration. The form of diarrhœa, occurring in this disease, shows that the incapacity for this transformation begins already in the intestinal canal. The severe symptoms of diminution or loss of consciousness show that the Ego-organization is driven out of the body and prevented from working properly. This is due to the fact that the albuminous substance cannot approach those mineralizing processes where the Ego-organization has power to work.

A further evidence lies in the fact that the evacuations carry the danger of infection. Here the tendency to destroy the inner forces of configuration shows itself highly enhanced.

Antimony preparations properly composed, and applied to these typhoid symptoms, prove an efficacious remedy. They divest the albuminous substance of the inherent forces to which it clings, and incline it to receive and incorporate the form-giving forces of the Ego-organization.

From the points of view that are so widespread and habitual to-day it will be said: Such conceptions as these about antimony are inexact. And they will emphasize in contrast the exact scientific nature of the methods of ordinary Chemistry. But in reality the chemical reactions of substances are no more significant for their action in the human organism than is the chemical composition of a paint for its manipulation by the artist. Undoubtedly the artist will do well to have some knowledge of the chemical starting-point from which he works. But the way in which he treats his materials as he paints the picture, is derived from quite another domain of principle and method. So it is with the therapeutic worker. Chemistry he can regard as an initial basis which has some real importance for him. But the mode of action of the substances within the human organism has nothing to do with this chemical domain. So long as we only see exactitude of method in the conclusions of ordinary Chemistry (including even its pharmaceutical branch), we annul the possibility of gaining true conceptions of what is taking place within the human body in the processes of healing.

CHAPTER XVII

Fundamental Knowledge of Substances

TO estimate the action of medicaments we must have an eye for the influences of forces which arise within the human organism, when a substance which shows certain characteristic activities while it is outside, is introduced into the body.

A classical instance is to be found in Formic Acid. Formic Acid occurs as a caustic inflammatory substance in the body of the ant. Here it appears as a secretion, which the organism of the animal must produce if it is to fulfil its proper activities. The life inherently consists in the secretory activity. Once it has been produced, the secretion no longer has a task within the organism; it must be excreted. The essence of a living organism lies not in its substances, but in its action. The organization is not a system of substances, it is an activity. A substance carries in it the stimulus and incitement to activity; once it has lost its stimulating power, it is no longer of importance to the organism.

In the human organism, too, formic acid is produced. Here, however, it has its importance. It serves the Ego-organization. The astral body separates out, from the organic substance, portions which tend to become lifeless. The Ego-organization needs this transition of organic substance to the lifeless state. But it is the process of transition which it needs, not the substance which is produced as a result. Once the substance which is on the way to the lifeless state has been produced, it becomes a burden to the organism. It must either then be separated out directly, or it must be dissolved in order to be eliminated indirectly.

Now if the solution of something which ought thus to be dissolved fails to take place, it will accumulate within the organism and may then constitute a foundation for conditions of gout or rheumatism. Here it is that the formic acid as it arises within the human organization plays its dissolving part. If the necessary amount of formic acid is produced, the organism will properly remove those products which are tending to the lifeless state. If the force to create formic acid is unduly weakened, rheumatic and gout-like conditions are the outcome. By introducing formic acid into the organism from outside, we can then come to its support, giving it what it is unable to create for itself.

We learn to recognize such modes of action by comparing one substance with another, with respect to the way in which they go on working in the human organism. Take Oxalic Acid for example. Under certain conditions it passes over into formic acid. The latter represents, in its influences and workings, a metamorphosis of oxalic acid. Oxalic acid is a secretion of the plant, as formic acid is of the animal nature. The creation of oxalic acid in the plant-organism is an activity analogous to that of formic acid in the animal. Which means, in other words, that the creation of oxalic acid corresponds to the domain of the Etheric and the creation of formic acid to the domain of the Astral. The diseases which reveal themselves in rheumatic and gout-like symptoms are to be ascribed to a deficient action of the astral body. Now the factors which in the case of gout and rheumatism proceed from the astral organism may also lie farther back, namely, in the etheric. Other morbid conditions will then present themselves. There will arise, not merely congestions of forces in the astral direction, to hinder and obstruct the Ego-organization, but hindrances in the etheric sphere which the astral organization itself is powerless to overcome. Such conditions reveal themselves in a sluggish action of the lower body, in the arrested functioning of liver and spleen, in the secretion of gall-stones and the like. If oxalic acid is administered in such cases, the activity of the etheric organism is correspondingly supported. Through oxalic acid the etheric body is strengthened; for the force of the Ego-organization is transformed by this acid into a force of the astral body, which acts in turn more vigorously on the etheric.

Taking our start from observations such as these, we can learn to recognize the wholesome and healing effects of various substances upon the body. In the plant, the physical activity is permeated by the etheric. In studying the plant, we learn to recognize how much can be attained by means of etheric activity. In the animal-astral organism, this activity is carried over to the astral. If, as etheric activity, it is too weak, it can then be strengthened by addition of the etheric activity proceeding from some plant product introduced into the body. The human organism is founded upon the underlying animal nature. Hence, *within certain limits*, where the interplay between the etheric body and the astral is concerned the same applies to the human organism as to the animal.

By the use of medicaments from the plant kingdom, we shall thus be able to remedy a disturbed relationship between the etheric and astral activities. But such medicaments will not

114

suffice when the physical, etheric, or astral organizations of man are disturbed in their mutual relation to the organization of the Ego. For the Ego-organization must apply its activity to processes which are tending to become mineral.

Accordingly, in the corresponding conditions of illness, mineral medicaments alone will be efficacious. To learn to know the remedial effects of a mineral substance, we must discover in what way and to what extent the substance can be disintegrated. For in the organism, the mineral introduced from outside must first be disintegrated, and then built up again in a new form by the organic forces proper to the body. In the disintegrative and reconstructive process any healing influence of the mineral must needs consist, and the outcome of it must lie in this direction: that a deficient action of the organism itself is taken over by the activity inherent in the medicament.

Take the case of an excessive menstruation. Here the power of the Ego-organization is enfeebled. It is expended one-sidedly in the preparation of blood. Too little is left of it for the power to absorb the blood within the organism. The path, which the forces in the organism that incline towards the lifeless realm should take, is unduly shortened. For they are working too vehemently and exhaust themselves half-way.

We can come to their assistance by administering calcium in some suitable combination. Calcium co-operates in the production and formation of the blood. The Ego is thus relieved of this sphere of its activity and enabled to devote its forces to the absorption of the blood.

CHAPTER XVIII

CURATIVE EURHYTHMY

WITHIN the domain of our therapeutic method, a special position is occupied by what we describe as Curative Eurhythmy. It is based on the Eurhythmy which was evolved—to begin with as a new form of Art—by Rudolf Steiner out of Anthroposophy.

The essential nature of the Art of Eurhythmy has often been described by Dr. Steiner, and indeed in its artistic form it has enjoyed wide recognition.

Eurhythmy is represented on the stage by the human being in movement; but it is not a form of dancing. This is evident already from the fact, that in Eurhythmy the movements of the arms and hands are above all important. Group movements enhance the whole effect, and the resulting picture on the stage gives a direct artistic impression.

All our movements are based on the inner nature of the human organization. From the same organization, in the earliest years of life, human speech proceeds. Now as in speech the spoken sound breaks forth from the inner constitution of man; so, with a real knowledge of this human constitution, we can derive from the single human being—or from the human beings in a group—movements which represent a true visible speech or visible song. These movements are as little arbitrary as speech itself. As in a spoken word an *O* cannot be pronounced where an *I* belongs, so in Eurhythmy only one kind of movement-gesture can appear for an *I* or for a C-sharp. Eurhythmy is thus a real and true manifestation of human nature, which can be evolved out of it, not indeed unconsciously like speech or song, but consciously by means of a true Knowledge of Man.

In the presentation of Eurhythmy we have human beings or groups of human beings in movement on the stage. The poem which is thus translated into visible speech is spoken simultaneously by a reciter. The audience hear the content of the poem and see it at the same time with their eyes. Or again, a piece of music is presented and appears at the same time as visible song in the movement-gestures of the performers.

Eurhythmy as a plastic Art of Movement constitutes a true extension of the sphere of the Fine Arts.

What has thus been discovered in the pure realm of Art can now be elaborated in two different directions. On the one hand it can be applied to Education. In the Waldorf School at Stuttgart, which was founded by Emil Molt and placed under the direction of Rudolf Steiner, educational Eurhythmy is done throughout the school in addition to the physical exercises or Gymnastics. The fact is, that in ordinary Gymnastics only the dynamics and statics of the physical body are developed. In Eurhythmy the full human being —body, soul, and spirit—goes out into movement. The growing child feels that this is so, and experiences the Eurhythmy exercises as a perfectly natural expression of his human nature—no less so than when in the earlier years of life he learned to speak.

The other application of Eurhythmy is therapeutic. The movement-gestures of the pure Art, and of educational Eurhythmy, modified so as to arise out of the morbid nature of man in the same way as they originally proceed from the healthy, give rise to a curative form of Eurhythmy.

The movements thus carried out react on the diseased organs. We observe how the movement outwardly executed is continued inwardly with a health-giving influence into the organs, provided always that the gesture of movement is accurately adapted to the organic disease. This method of influencing the human being through movement, affecting him as it does in body, soul, and Spirit, works more intensely into the inner nature of the patient than any other system of therapeutic movement.

For this very reason, Curative Eurhythmy can never become an affair for amateurs. On no account must it be regarded or applied as such.

The Curative Eurhythmist, who must be well trained in a knowledge of the human organization, may only work in connection with the qualified Doctor. All amateurish performances in this direction can but lead to ill results. It is only on the basis of a true and thorough diagnosis that the Curative Eurhythmy exercises can properly be done.

The results of Curative Eurhythmy, as applied in practice, are indeed such as to warrant its description as an exceedingly beneficial element within the therapeutic method explained in this book.

CHAPTER XIX

CHARACTERISTIC CASES

IN this chapter we shall describe a number of cases from the practice of the Clinical and Therapeutic Institute at Arlesheim. They will show how with the help of a knowledge of spiritual man, we may try to gain an exhaustive and penetrating picture of the diseased condition, so much so that the very diagnosis teaches us the remedy to be applied. Fundamental to this is a perception which recognizes the process of illness and of healing as a single cycle. The illness begins with an irregularity in the constitution of the human organism, with respect to its several parts which have been described in this book. It has already reached a certain stage when the patient is received for treatment. Our object must now be to bring about a reversal of all the processes which have taken place in the organism since the beginning of the illness, so that they return to their starting-point, and we arrive at length at the condition of health in which the organism was to begin with. A cyclic process of this kind, returning in itself, cannot be accomplished without the organism as a whole suffering some loss in forces of growth —forces equivalent to those which the human organism needs during childhood in order to enlarge its volume. The medicaments must therefore be so composed as not only to bring the diseased process back to its starting-point, but to supplement once more the decreasing vitality. To some extent this latter influence must be left to dietary treatment; but as a general rule, in the more serious cases of illness, the body is not in a condition to evolve sufficient vitality in the assimilation of its food. Thus the therapeutic treatment proper will also have to be so constituted as to give the organism the necessary support in this respect. In the typical remedies supplied by our Clinical and Therapeutic Institutes, this provision has been made throughout. Hence it will only be realized on a closer inspection why a given preparation contains such and such constituents. In estimating the course of the disease, not only the localized morbid process, but the changes suffered by the organism as a whole must be considered, and included in the returning process of the cure. How this is to be conceived in detail will be shown by the individual cases which we shall now describe. We shall then continue the more general considerations.

First Case

A woman patient, twenty-six years old. The whole personality reveals an extraordinarily un-stable condition. It is clear from the patient's appearance that that part of the organism which we have here called the astral body is in an ex-cessive state of activity. One observes that the Ego-organization cannot master the astral body save in a very deficient way. As soon as the patient begins to do some work, the astral body is imme-diately in a state of agitation. The Ego-organiza-tion tries to make itself felt, but is constantly pushed back again, with the result that whenever she tries to work, a rise of temperature occurs. The regular activity of digestion in the human being is in the highest degree dependent on a normal Ego-organization. The powerlessness of this patient's Ego-organization accordingly finds expression in an obstinate state of constipation. The migraine-like conditions and vomiting from which she suffers are another consequence of this disturbance in the digestive activity. In sleep her weak Ego-organization appears to give rise to a deficient organic activity from below upwards, and the out-breathing process is impaired. Thus there is an excessive accumulation of carbonic acid in the system during sleep. Organically this finds expression in palpitation on awakening, psychically in a sense of terror: the patient will suddenly cry out. Examination of her bodily condition reveals nothing else than a lack of those forces which bring about a regular connection of the astral, etheric, and physical bodies. Owing to the excessive activity of the astral body in itself, too little of its powers can flow over into the physical and the etheric. The latter, therefore, have remained too delicate and tender in their development during the period of growth. This finds expression in the patient's slight and feeble build, and also in the fact that she complains of frequent pains in the back. Such pains arise, because in the activity of the spinal cord the Ego-organization above all must make itself strongly felt. The patient tells of frequent and continual dreams. The reason is that the astral body, separated in sleep from the physical and the etheric, gives vent to its own excessive activity.

We therefore take our start from the fact that the Ego-organization needs to be strengthened, and the over-activity of the astral body simultaneously lowered. The former object is attained by selecting a remedy that can assist the weakened Ego-organization in the digestive tract. Such a remedy is to be found in copper. Applied in the form of a copper ointment to the region of the loins, it has a strengthening effect on the evolution of inner warmth, which, proceeding from the Ego-organization, is deficient. The good effect of this is observed in a reduction of the abnormal activity of the heart and a cessation of the feeling of terror. The excessive activity of the astral body in itself is combated by exceedingly minute doses of lead taken internally. Lead draws the astral body together and awakens in it the forces to unite more intensely with the physical body and the etheric. (Lead poisoning, in fact, represents an over-intense union of the astral with the etheric and physical bodies, so that the latter are made subject to excessive processes of disintegration.)

The patient recovered visibly under this treatment. Her unstable condition gave way to a certain inner firmness and assurance. Her life of feeling, recovering from its disrupted state, grew inwardly calm and contented. The constipation and the pains in the back disappeared, likewise the migraine conditions and the headaches. The patient's power of work was restored.

Second Case

A man of forty-eight years. He had been a robust child with a healthy and vigorous inner life. During the war, as he informed us, he had undergone a five months' treatment for nephritis and been discharged as cured. Married at the age of thirty-five, he had five healthy children; a sixth child died at birth. At the age of thirty-three, as a consequence of mental overwork, he began to suffer from depression, weariness, and apathy. These conditions grew more and more intense. At the same time he began to feel mentally and spiritually at a loss. He is confronted by endless questions and misgivings, in which his profession (that of a schoolmaster) appears to him in a negative light, nor can he bring forth anything positive with which to meet his troubles. This morbid condition reveals an astral body having too little affinity with the etheric and physical, and in its own nature immobile. The physical and etheric bodies are thus enabled to assert their own inherent qualities. The feeling of the etheric not being rightly united with the astral body gives rise to states of depression, while the deficient union with the physical produces fatigue and apathy. That the patient is mentally and spiritually at a loss, is due to the fact that the astral body cannot make proper use of the physical and the etheric. Consistently with all this, his sleep is good; for the astral body has little connection with the etheric and physical. For the same reason he has great difficulty in waking up; the astral body is loath to enter into the physical. It is only in the evening, when the physical and etheric

126

bodies are tired, that their normal union with the astral begins to take place. Thus the patient does not become properly awake until the evening.

This whole condition indicates that it is necessary first of all to strengthen the astral body in its activity—a thing that can always be attained by giving arsenic internally in the form of a mineral water. After a time under such treatment the human being is seen to gain more command over his body. The connection between the astral and the etheric is strengthened; the depression, apathy, and fatigue are made to cease. But the physical body also, which during the prolonged defective union with the astral has grown sluggish and immobile, must be assisted. This is done by giving phosphorus in weak doses. Phosphorus supports the Ego-organization, enabling it to overcome the resistance of the physical body. Rosemary baths are applied to open a way out for the accumulated products of metabolism. A curative eurhythmy treatment re-establishes the harmony of the several members of the organization (nerves-and-senses system, rhythmic system, motor and metabolic system), impaired as it is by the long inaction of the astral body. Finally, by giving the patient elder-flower tea, the metabolism, which has gradually become sluggish owing to the inactivity of the astral body, is restored to a normal condition.

127

We had the satisfaction of observing a complete cure in this case.

Third Case

This patient was a musician, thirty-one years old, who visited our Clinic during a concert tour. He was suffering from a severe inflammatory and functional disorder of the urinary organs; catarrhal symptoms, fever, excessive bodily fatigue, general weakness, and incapacity for work.

The past history of the patient showed that he had repeatedly suffered from similar conditions. Investigation of his spiritual condition revealed a hypersensitive and excessively tender astral body. The quick susceptibility of the physical and etheric body to catarrhal and inflammatory conditions is due to this. Already as a child, the patient had a weak physical body, badly nurtured and supported by the astral. Hence measles, scarlet fever, chicken-pox, whooping-cough, and frequent affections of the throat. At the age of fourteen there was an inflammation of the urethra, which recurred at the age of twenty-nine in conjunction with cystitis. At the age of eighteen, pneumonia and pleurisy; at twenty-nine, pleurisy again, following on an attack of influenza; and at the age of thirty, catarrhal inflammation of the frontal sinus. There is also a perpetual tendency to catarrhal conjunctivitis.

128

During the two months which he spent at the Clinic, the patient's temperature curve rose at first to 102, after which it descended, but only to rise again a fortnight later. It then oscillated between 98.6 and 96.8, occasionally rising above 98.6 and going down even as low as 95. This temperature curve gives a clear picture of the changing moods in the Ego-organization. Such a curve arises when the effects of the semi-conscious contents of the Ego-organization find expression in the warmth-processes of the physical and etheric bodies, without being reduced to a normal rhythm by the astral. In this patient, the whole power of action of the astral body was concentrated on the rhythmic system, where it found expression in his artistic talent. The other systems no longer received their proper share.

As a significant result of this, the patient suffers from severe fatigue and insomnia during the summer. In the summer season, considerable demands are made upon the astral body by the outer world, and its power of inward activity is thereby reduced. The forces of the physical and etheric body become predominant. This manifests itself, in the patient's general sense of life, as an intense feeling of fatigue. At the same time the weakened power and initiative of the astral body hinder its separation from the physical:

hence the insomnia. The deficient severance of the astral body from the etheric finds expression in unpleasant and exciting dreams, arising from the sensitiveness of the etheric body to the lesions in the physical organism. Characteristically, the dreams symbolize these lesions in images of mutilated human beings. Their terrifying aspect is simply their natural quality and emphasis of feeling. As a consequence of the astral body functioning deficiently in the metabolic system, there is a tendency to constipation. And owing to the independence of the etheric body, which is too little influenced by the astral, the albumen received as food cannot be completely transformed from vegetable and animal albumen into human. Hence albumen is excreted in the urine: the albumen reaction is positive. Moreover, when the astral body is functioning deficiently, processes will arise in the physical body which are really foreign processes in the human organism. Such processes express themselves in the formation of pus, which represents, as it were, an extra-human process within the human being. Thus in the sediment of the urine we find pure pus. But this formation of pus is accompanied by a parallel process in the life of the soul. The astral body of the patient is no less deficient psychically in assimilating the experiences of life, than physically in assimilating

130

the substances of food. While extra-human substance-formations are produced in the shape of pus, mental and psychic contents of an extra-human character arise at the same time—as a keen interest in abnormal relationships of life, forebodings, premonitions, and the like.

We therefore set out to bring a balancing, purifying, and strengthening influence to bear upon the astral body. The Ego-organization being very much alive, its activity could be used, in a manner of speaking, as a carrier of the influences of healing. Now the Ego-organization, which is focussed on the external world, is most readily approached by influences whose direction is from without inward. This is attained by the use of bandages or compresses. We first apply a compress of *melilotus*, a remedy which works upon the astral body in such a way as to improve the balance and distribution of its forces, counteracting their one-sided concentration on the rhythmic system. Naturally the compresses must not be applied to those portions of the body where the rhythmic system is especially concentrated. We applied it to the organs where the metabolic and motor systems have their main centre. Head-bandages we avoided, because the changing mood of the Ego-organization, proceeding from the head, would only have paralysed the remedial influence. For the melilotus to take effect, it was also necessary to assist the astral body and Ego-organization, drawing them together and tightening their union. This we sought to do by an added constituent containing oxalic acid, derived from *radix bardanae*. Oxalic acid works in such a way as to transform the activity of the Ego-organization into that of the astral body.

In addition, we administered internal remedies in very minute doses with the object of bringing the secretions into a regular connection with the influences of the astral body. The secretions which are directed from the head-system, we tried to normalize by means of potassium sulphate. Those that depend upon the metabolic system in the narrower sense of the word, we sought to influence by potassium carbonate. The secretion of urine we regulated by the use of *teucrium*. We therefore gave a medicament consisting of equal parts of potassium sulphate, potassium carbonate, and teucrium. The whole of this treatment had to reckon with a very unstable balance in the organism as a whole: physically, psychically, and spiritually. Thus we had to provide for physical rest by keeping the patient in bed, and for spiritual equilibrium by promoting quiet of mind and soul. This alone made possible the proper interpenetration of the various remedies.

On the completion of the cure, the patient was restored to bodily strength and vigour, and was mentally in good condition. With a constitution so unstable it goes without saying that some external disturbance may bring about a recurrence of one disorder or another. In such a case it is essential to a complete cure that violent disturbances should be avoided.

Fourth Case

A child, who was brought into our Clinic twice, first at the age of four, and then at the age of five and a half years; also the mother of the child, and the mother's sister. Diagnosis led from the disease of the child to that of the mother and of her sister. As to the child itself, we received the following information: It was a twin-child, born six weeks too early. The other twin died in the last stage of embryonal life. At the age of six weeks, the child was taken ill, screaming to an unusual extent, and was transferred to hospital where they diagnosed pylorospasmus. The child was nourished by a nurse and also artificially. At the age of eight months it left the hospital. On the first day after arrival home the child had convulsions, which were repeated every day for the next two months. During the attacks the child became stiff, with the eyes distorted. The attacks were preceded by fear and crying. The child squinted with the right eye, and vomited before the attack began. At the age of two and a half years there was another attack lasting five hours. The child was stiff and lay there as though dead. At the age of four there was an attack lasting half an hour. According to the report we received, this was the first attack which was seen to be accompanied by fever symptoms. After the attacks that had followed directly on the return from hospital, the parents had noticed a paralysis of the right arm and the right leg. At two and a half the child made the first attempt to walk, but was only able to step out with the left leg, dragging the right after it. The right arm, too, remained without volition.

Our first concern was to determine the condition of the child with respect to the several members of the human organization. This was attempted independently of the external complex of symptoms. We found a severe atrophy of the etheric body, which in certain parts received the influence of the astral body only to a very slight extent. The region of the right breast was as though paralysed in the etheric body. On the other hand, there was a kind of hypertrophy of the astral body in the region of the stomach. The next thing was to establish the relation between this diagnosis and the outer complex of symptoms. There could be no doubt that the stomach was powerfully engaged by the astral body in the process of digestion. At the same time, owing to the paralysed condition of the etheric body, the digestive process became congested and held up in its passage from the intestinal tract into the lymphatic vessels. Hence the blood was under-nourished. We thus attached great importance to the symptoms of nausea and vomiting. Convulsions always occur when the etheric body becomes atrophied and the astral gains a direct influence over the physical without the mediation of the etheric. Such a condition existed in the highest degree in this little child. Moreover, if, as in this case, the condition becomes permanent during the period of growth, those processes which normally prepare the motor system to receive the Will fail to take place. This showed itself in the impotence of the child on the right side of the body.

We had now to relate the condition of the child with that of the mother. The latter was thirty-seven years old when she came to us. At the age of thirteen, she told us, she had already reached her present size. She had bad teeth at an early age, and had suffered in childhood from articular rheumatism. She also said that she had been inclined to rickets. Menstruation began comparatively soon. At the age of sixteen, according to her account, she had had a disease of the kidneys, and she told of cramp-like conditions from which she had suffered in this connection. At twenty-five she had constipation owing to cramp in the sphinctor ani, which had to be artificially dilated. Even now she suffered from cramp during evacuation.

Diagnosis by direct observation (without drawing any conclusions from this complex of symptoms) revealed a condition extraordinarily similar to that of the child, with this difference, that everything appeared in a far milder form. We must bear in mind that the human etheric body has its special period of development between the change of teeth and puberty. In the mother this fact expressed itself as follows: With their deficient strength, the available forces of the etheric body enabled growth to take place only until puberty. At puberty the special development of the astral body begins. At this stage the patient's astral body, being hypertrophied, overwhelmed the etheric body and took hold of the physical organization too intensely. This showed itself in the arrest of growth at the thirteenth year. The patient was, however, by no means small; on the contrary, she was very big. In effect, the growth forces of the etheric body, small as they were, had been unhindered by the astral body, and had thus brought about a large expansion of the physical body in volume. But they had not been able to enter regularly into the functions of the physical body; hence the appearance of articular rheumatism, and at a later stage, cramp and convulsions. Owing to the weakness of the etheric body there was an abnormally strong influence of the astral body on the physical. Now this influence is a disintegrating one. In the normal development of man's life, it is balanced and held in check by the upbuilding forces during sleep, when the astral body is severed from the physical and the etheric. If, as in this case, the etheric body is too weak, the result is an excess of disintegration. Thus the bad condition of the patient's teeth had made the first stopping necessary at the early age of twelve. Moreover, if great demands are made on the forces of the etheric body as in pregnancy, on every such occasion the condition of the teeth grows worse. The weakness of the etheric body with respect to its connection with the astral was also shown by the frequency of the patient's dreams, and by the sound sleep which she enjoyed in spite of all irregularities. Again, when the etheric body is weakened, foreign processes are apt to take place in the physical body which the etheric cannot master. Such processes revealed themselves in the urine as albumen, isolated hyaline casts, and salts.

Very remarkable was the relation of the disease-processes in the mother with those from which her sister was suffering. As to the composition of the members of the human being, diagnosis revealed almost exactly the same: a feebly working etheric body and hence a preponderance of the astral. The astral body was, however, weaker than that of the former patient. Accordingly, menstruation had begun too soon as in the former case, but instead of inflammatory conditions she had only suffered from pains due to an irritation of the organs, notably the articulations. In the articulations the etheric body must be peculiarly active if the vitality is to go on in the normal way. If the activity of the etheric body is weak, that of the physical body will predominate—a fact which appeared in this case in the swollen joints and in chronic arthritis. The weakness of the astral body, which did not work enough in the subjective feeling of the patient, was indicated by her liking for sweet dishes. Sweet food enhances the conscious feeling of the astral body. When the weak astral body is exhausted at the end of the day, then, if the weakness persists, the pains will increase in intensity. Thus the patient complained of increased pain in the evening.

The connection between the morbid conditions of these three patients points to the generation preceding that of the two sisters, and more especially to the grandmother of the child. It is here that the real cause must be sought for. The disordered equilibrium between the astral and etheric bodies in all three patients can only have arisen from a similar condition in the grandmother of the child. The irregularity must, in fact, have been due to an under-development, by the astral and etheric bodies of the grandmother, of the embryonal organs of nourishment—especially the allantois. There must have been a deficient development of the allantois in all three patients. We determined this to begin with by purely spiritual scientific methods. The physical allantois, passing into the spiritual realm, is metamorphosed into the strength and vigour of the forces of the astral body. A degenerated allantois gives rise to a lessened efficiency of the astral body, which will express itself especially in all the motor organs. Such was the case in all three patients. It is indeed possible to recognize, from the constitution of the astral body, that of the allantois. From this it will be seen that our reference to the preceding generation was the result, not of an adventurous and fancied drawing of conclusions, but of real spiritual-scientific observation.

To anyone who is irritated by this fact, we would say that our statements here are not inspired by any love of paradox. We simply desire that knowledge, which has in fact come into being, shall be withheld from no one. Conceptions of heredity will always remain dark and mystical as they are to-day, so long as science shrinks from recognizing the metamorphosis from the physical to the spiritual which takes place in the sequence of the generations.

Therapeutically, this insight could of course only lead us to perceive the right starting-point for a healing process. Had not our attention thus been drawn to the hereditary aspect—had we simply observed the irregularity in the condition of the astral and etheric bodies—we should have used remedies apt to influence these two members of the human being. But such remedies would have been ineffective in this case, for the disorder —continuing, as it did, through the successive generations—was too deep-seated to be restored to a normal condition within the etheric and astral bodies themselves. In a case like this, one must work on the organization of the Ego. Here it is that one must bring to bear all those influences which relate to a harmonizing and strengthening of the etheric and astral bodies. To do so, one must gain access to the Ego-organization, as it were, through intensified sensory stimuli. (Sensory stimuli work upon the Ego-organization.)

For the child, we attempted this in the following way. We bandaged the right hand with a 5 per cent. iron pyrites ointment. Simultaneously we massaged the left half of the head with ointment of *amanita cæsarea*. Externally applied, pyrites— a compound of iron and sulphur—has the effect of stimulating the Ego-organization to make the astral body more alive and increase its affinity to the etheric. The amanita substance, with its peculiar contents of organized nitrogen, gives rise to an influence proceeding from the head, which, working through the Ego-organization, makes the etheric body more alive and increases its affinity to the astral. This treatment was supplemented by Curative Eurhythmy, which brings the Ego-organization as such into a quickened action. The healing processes externally applied are thus carried right into the depths of the system. Initiated in this way, the healing process was then intensified, with remedies contrived to make the astral and etheric bodies especially sensitive to the influence of the Ego-organization. In rhythmic succession day after day, we gave baths with a decoction of *solidago*, massaged the back with a decoction of *stellaria media*, and gave internally a tea prepared from willow-bark (which affects the receptivity especially of the astral body) and *stannum* 0.001 (which makes the etheric body especially receptive). We also gave weak doses of poppy juice, to make the disordered organization as a whole less assertive, and more susceptible to the influences of healing.

In the mother's case, the latter kind of treatment was mainly adopted, since the inherited forces— one generation farther back—had not yet worked to so great an extent. The same applied to the sister of the mother.

While the child was still with us in the Clinic, we observed that it became more easily directed and the general psychological condition was improved. It grew far more obedient. Movements which it had done very clumsily, it now accomplished with greater skill. Subsequently the aunt reported that a great change had taken place in the child. It had grown quieter, and the excess of involuntary movements had decreased. The child is now sufficiently adroit to be able to play by itself, and in the inner life of soul, the former obstinacy has disappeared.

Fifth Case

A woman patient, twenty-six years old, who came to our Clinic suffering from the serious consequences of influenza and catarrhal pneumonia which she had undergone in 1918. This had been preceded in 1917 by pleurisy. Since the influenza she had never properly recovered. In 1920 she was very much emaciated and in a feeble condition, with slight temperature and nocturnal perspiration. Soon after the influenza she had begun to suffer from pains in the back which grew increasingly till the end of 1920. Then, with a violent increase in the pain, curvature of the spine became apparent in the lumbar region. At the same time there was a swelling of the right forefinger. A rest cure was said to have considerably lessened the pains in the back.

When the patient came to us, she was suffering from a gravitation abscess on the right thigh. Her body was distended and she had slight ascites. There were catarrhal noises over the apices of both lungs. Digestion and appetite were good. The urine was concentrated, with traces of albumen.

Spiritual-scientific investigation revealed a hypersensitiveness of the astral body and the Ego-organization. An abnormality of this kind expresses itself to begin with in the etheric body, which evolves, in place of the etheric functions proper, an etheric impress of the astral functions. Now the astral functions are disintegrative. Thus the general vitality and the normal process in the physical organs were necessarily atrophied. Such a condition is always accompanied by processes to some extent extra-human, taking place within the human organism. Hence the gravitation abscess, the lumbar pains, the distended abdomen, the catarrhal symptoms in the lungs, and also the deficient assimilation of albumen. The therapeutic treatment must therefore seek to lower the sensitiveness of the astral body and the Ego-organization. This may be done by administering silica, which always strengthens the active inherent forces against undue sensitiveness. In this case we gave powdered silica in the food and in an enema treatment. We also diverted the excessive sensitiveness by applying mustard plasters to the loins. The effect of this depends upon the fact that it induces sensitiveness of its own accord, thus relieving the astral body and Ego-organization to some extent of theirs. By a process which damps down the over-sensitiveness of the astral body in the digestive tract, we contrived to divert the astral activity in this region to the etheric body where it ought normally to be. To this end we gave minute doses of copper and *carbo animalis*. The possibility that the etheric body might shrink from the normal activity of digestion, to which it was unaccustomed, was countered by administering pancreatic fluid.

The gravitation abscess was punctured several

times. Large quantities of pus were evacuated by aspiration, the abscess became very much reduced and the distended stomach decreased at the same time. The formation of pus grew continuously less and came to an end. While it was still flowing we were surprised one day by a renewed rise in temperature. This was not inexplicable to us, since, with the above-described constitution of the astral body, even small psychological excitements could easily give rise to fever. But the possibility of accounting for a rise in temperature in such cases in no way lessens the very serious effect of it when it occurs. For under these conditions, such a fever is a most deadly mediator for a far-reaching entry of the disintegrative processes into the system. One must provide at once for a strengthening of the etheric body, which will then paralyse the harmful effects of the astral. We gave silver injections at a high potency and the fever declined.

The patient left the Clinic with a twenty pounds' increase in weight, and considerably stronger. We are well aware that an after-treatment will be necessary in this case to make the cure a lasting one.

*   *   *   *

With the cases hitherto described, we wished to

characterize the principles whereby we seek to find the remedies directly out of the diagnosis. For the sake of clear and vivid illustration we selected cases where it was necessary to proceed along very individual lines. But we have also prepared typical remedies, applicable to typical diseases. We will now deal with a few cases where such typical medicaments were applied.

Sixth Case. *Treatment of Hay Fever*

We received a patient with severe hay fever symptoms. He had suffered from it already in his childhood and was in his fortieth year when he came to us for treatment. Against this morbid condition we have our preparation " Gencydo," which we applied in this case in the season (the month of May) when the disease affected the patient in its most violent form. We gave him the injections and also the local treatment, painting the interior of the nose with Gencydo fluid. At a time of year when in former years he had still had to suffer severely from the hay fever symptoms, there was a marked improvement. He then undertook a journey, whence he reported that he felt incomparably better than in former years. In the hay fever season of the next year, he was travelling again from America to Europe and had only a far slighter attack. Our repeated treatment during

146

that year put him in a very bearable condition. To make the cure a thorough one he was treated again the following year, though there was no proper attack. In the fourth year the patient himself described his condition in the following words: " In the spring of 1923, I again began the treatment, as I was expecting fresh attacks. I found my nasal mucous membranes far less sensitive than before. I had to spend my time working in the midst of flowering grasses and pollen-producing trees. I also had to ride all through the summer along hot and dusty roads. But with the exception of a single day, no symptoms of hay fever occurred the whole summer, and I have every reason to believe that on that day it was an ordinary cold, and not an attack of hay fever. For thirty-five years this was the first time that I could stay and work unhindered in an environment where in former years I suffered indescribably."

Seventh Case. Treatment of Sclerosis

A woman patient, sixty-one years old, came to our Clinic with sclerosis and albuminuria. Her immediate condition was the sequel of an attack of influenza, with slight fever and disturbances of the stomach and intestines. She had not felt well again since the influenza. She complained of difficult breathing on awakening, attacks of vertigo, and a knocking or beating sensation in the head, ears, and hands, which was especially troublesome on awakening, but occurred also when she walked or climbed uphill. Her sleep was good. There was a tendency to constipation and the urine contained albumen. Her blood pressure was 185 mm.

We took our start from the sclerosis, which was noticeable in the over-activity of the astral body. The physical and etheric bodies were unable to receive into themselves the full activity of the astral. In such a case, an extra activity of the astral body remains over, which the physical and etheric fail to re-absorb. Now the normal and firm composure of the human organization is only possible when this re-absorption is complete. Otherwise, as in the case of our patient, the non-absorbed remnant will make itself felt in attacks of vertigo and subjective sensory illusions—knocking noises and the like. Also the non-absorbed portion seizes hold of the substances received as food, and forces certain processes upon them before they have penetrated into the normal metabolism. This became apparent in the tendency to constipation, in the secretion of albumen, and in the stomach and intestinal disorders. The blood pressure is increased in such a case because the over-activity of the astral body heightens also

148

the activity of the Ego, which activity reveals itself in the high blood pressure.

We treated the case mainly with our " Scleron " remedy, which we only supplemented with very minute doses of belladonna, in order to meet the attacks of vertigo momentarily as well, when they occurred. We gave elder-flower tea to help the digestion and regulated the action of the bowels by enemas and laxative tea. We ordered a saltless diet because salts will rapidly assist sclerosis. A comparatively quick improvement was the result. The attacks of vertigo receded, likewise the beating sensations. The blood pressure went down to 112. The patient's subjective feeling visibly improved. During the subsequent year the sclerosis made no further progress. At the end of a year the patient came to us again with the same symptoms in a lesser degree. A similar treatment brought about a further improvement, and now, after a lapse of considerable time, it is evident that the sclerosis is producing no further degeneration of the organism. The external symptoms characteristic of sclerosis are on the decline, and the rapid ageing process by which the patient had been seized exists no longer.

Eighth Case. A Treatment of Goitre

A woman patient, who came to us in the thirty-fourth year of her life. She is the very type of a

human being whose whole inner life is strongly
influenced by a certain heaviness, an internal
crumbling, of the physical body. Every word she
utters seems to cost her an effort. Extremely
characteristic is the concavity in the shape of her
face; the root of the nose seems to be held back,
as it were, within the organism. She tells us that
she was delicate and sickly even as a child. The
only proper disease she underwent was a slight
attack of measles. She was always pale and
suffered from fatigue and a bad appetite. She was
sent from one doctor to another, and the following
were diagnosed in succession: Apex pulmonary
catarrh, gastric catarrh, anæmia. In her own
consciousness, the patient feels that she is ill not
so much in body as in soul.

Having given this extract of her past history,
we will now indicate the spiritual-scientific diagnosis, in connection with which all other things
will then be examined.

The patient reveals a highly atonic condition of
the astral body. The Ego-organization is thus
thrown back, as it were, from the physical and
etheric bodies. The whole life of consciousness is
permeated in a delicate way by a dim, sleepy
condition. The physical body is exposed to the
processes arising from the substances it receives
from outside, which substances are thus trans-

formed into parts of the human organization. The etheric body is too much damped and lowered in its own coherent vitality by the Ego and astral body. Hence the inner sensations—namely, the general sense of life and the sense of the statics of the body—become far too strong and vivid, while on the other hand the life of the external senses is too dim. All the bodily functions thus have to take a course whereby they come into disharmony with one another. Inevitably the feeling arises in the patient that she cannot hold the functions of her body together with her own Ego. This appears to her as weakness, powerlessness of soul; and hence she says she is more ill in soul than in body.

If the weakness of the Ego and astral body increase, morbid conditions will necessarily arise in various parts of the body, as indicated by the different diagnoses. Powerlessness of the Ego comes to expression in irregularities of glands, such as the thyroid and the suprarenal; also in disorders of the stomach and intestinal system. All this is to be expected in the patient and does in fact occur. Her goitre and the condition of her stomach and intestinal system agree entirely with the spiritual-scientific diagnosis. Most characteristic is the following: Owing to the powerlessness of the Ego and astral body, part of the required sleep is absolved during the waking life. Hence her sleep is lighter than in the normal human being. To the patient herself this appears as an obstinate insomnia. In close connection with this, she has a sense of easily falling asleep and easily awakening. Again, she thinks she has many dreams; they are not, however, real dreams but mixtures of dreams and waking impressions. Thus they do not remain in her memory and are not at all powerfully exciting, for her excitability is lowered.

In the inner organs the powerlessness of the Ego finds expression first of all in the lungs. Apex pulmonary catarrhs are in reality always a manifestation of a weak Ego-organization. The metabolism not being fully accomplished by the Ego expresses itself in rheumatism. Subjectively these things come to expression in the patient's general state of fatigue. Menstruation began at the age of fourteen. The weak Ego-organization cannot supply a sufficient unfolding of forces to repress and restrain the menstrual process once it is in flow. Now the work of the Ego in this act of restraint comes to conscious sensation through the nerves that enter the spinal cord in the region of the sacrum. Nerves insufficiently permeated by the currents of the Ego-organization and astral body are generally painful. Thus the patient complains of lumbar pains during menstruation.

All this led us to a therapeutic treatment in the following manner: We have discovered that *colchicum autumnale* has a powerfully stimulating action on the astral body, notably on the part that corresponds to the organization of the neck and head. Hence we apply *colchicum autumnale* to all those diseases which have their most important symptom in goitre. Accordingly we gave the patient five drops of our colchicum preparation three times a day. The goitre swelling receded and the patient felt much relieved. When the astral body is thus strengthened, it mediates for a better functioning of the Ego-organism, so that remedies which can work upon the organs of digestion and reproduction receive their proper power in the organism. We administered worm-wood as an enema treatment, mingling it with oil, since oil gives rise to an excitation in the digestive tract. With this remedy we attained a considerable improvement.

We hold that the above treatment can develop its favourable influence especially about the thirty-fifth year of life, for at this age the Ego-organization has a peculiarly strong affinity to the rest of the organism and can readily be stimulated and called to life, even when weak in its own nature. The patient was thirty-four years old when she came to us.

Ninth Case. Migraine Conditions in the Menopause

This patient comes to us at the age of fifty-five. She tells that she was a slender and delicate child. During childhood she had measles, scarlet fever, chicken-pox, whooping cough, and mumps. Menstruation began at the age of fourteen to fifteen. The hæmorrhages were unusually intense and painful from the outset. At the age of forty she underwent a total extirpation owing to a tumour in the abdomen. She also reports that she suffered since the age of thirty-five, every three or four weeks, from a migraine-headache lasting three days. At forty-six this was intensified, developing into a regular disease of the head which went on for three days and involved even a loss of consciousness.

The spiritual-scientific diagnosis of her present condition is as follows: General weakness of the Ego-organization, which proves unable sufficiently to tone down the activity of the etheric body. Hence the vegetative organic activity spreads itself out over the head-system—the system of nerves and senses—to a far higher degree than is the case when the Ego-organization is normal. This diagnosis is corroborated by certain symptoms, for example, the frequent desire for urination. This is due to the fact that the astral body which regulates the secretion of the kidneys is normally developed, while the Ego-organization, which should normally hold it in check, is not strong enough. Another symptom is the long time she takes to fall asleep and her tiredness on awakening. The astral body has a difficulty in leaving the physical and etheric, for the Ego is not strong enough in drawing it away. And when she has awakened, the vital activity, working on as an after-effect from sleep, gives her a feeling of fatigue owing to the weakness of the Ego. A third symptom is to be found in the fewness of her dreams; the pictures which the Ego-organization can stamp upon the astral body are but feeble and cannot express themselves as vivid dreams.

These perceptions led to the following therapeutic treatment: It was necessary to make way for the Ego-organization to enter into the physical and etheric bodies. We did this by compresses with a 2 per cent. salt-of-sorrel solution on the forehead in the evening; bandages with a 7 per cent. solution of *urtica dioica* on the abdomen in the morning; and bandages with a 20 per cent. solution of lime-tree flower on the feet at noon. The object was in the first place to weaken and tone down the vital activity during the night. This was brought about by the oxalic salt, which exercises, within the organism, the function of suppressing an excessive vital activity. In the morning our care was to help the Ego-organization to find its way into the physical body. This is done by stimulating the circulation of the blood. The influence of iron, contained in the influence of the nettle (*urtica dioica*), was applied for this purpose. Finally, it was desirable to assist the penetration of the physical body with the Ego-organization during the rest of the day. This was done by the downward-drawing influence of the lime-tree flower bandages at noon.

We have already referred to the headaches to which the patient had become subject, with their intensification at the forty-sixth year of life. We had to relate these headaches to the cessation of the menses on extirpation; their intensification with symptoms of unconsciousness must indeed be regarded as a compensatory symptom of the menopause. We first tried to effect an improvement by the use of antimony, which would certainly have worked if it had been a question of the general metabolism, regulated by the organization of the Ego.

There was, however, no improvement. This showed us that the relatively independent part of the Ego-organization which primarily regulates the organs of reproduction was in reality concerned. For the treatment of this, we see a specific in the root of *potentilla tormentilla* at a very high dilution; and indeed this remedy had the desired effect.

CHAPTER XX

WE shall now describe, and explain the remedial value of a few of our typical medicaments, some of which have been placed upon the market. They are adapted to the typical forms of disease; and in so far as a morbid condition is typical, our medicament will represent the necessary means to bring about a therapeutic action in the sense of the explanations of this book. From this point of view a number of our medicaments will be described.

1. "*Scleron*"

Scleron consists of metallic lead, honey, and sugar. Lead works upon the organism in such a way as to stimulate the disintegrating action of the Ego-organization. If we introduce it into the organism where this action is deficient, it will therefore stimulate it, if administered in sufficiently strong doses. If the doses are excessive, hypertrophy of the Ego-organization is the result, and the body disintegrates more than it can build. In Sclerosis the Ego-organization becomes too weak, and its own disintegrating action is insufficient. Hence disintegration begins to take place by the agency of the astral body alone. The products of disintegration fall out of the totality of the organism, and give rise to a thickening of the organs, consisting in salt-like substances. Lead, given in proper doses, brings the disintegrating action back into the Ego-organization. The products of disintegration no longer remain as a hardening within the body, but are driven outward. There can, indeed, be no cure of Sclerosis except by enabling the salt-forming processes, which otherwise remain in the body, to find their way out.

By means of lead we thus determine the *direction* of the processes of the Ego-organization. But it is necessary to keep these processes fluid, as it were, in their further course. This is done by the admixture of honey. Honey enables the Ego-organization to exercise the necessary dominion over the astral body. It deprives the astral body of that relative independence which it acquires in Sclerosis. Sugar works upon the Ego-organization directly, strengthening it in its own nature. Our remedy, therefore, has the following effect: The lead itself works disintegratingly, not like the astral body, but like the Ego-organization. The honey transfers the disintegrating action of the astral body to the Ego-organization, and the sugar puts the Ego-organization in a condition to fulfil its specific task.

The initial stages of Sclerosis may be observed to express themselves in psychological symptoms. The human being loses his quickness and readiness of thought and his precise command of memory. Applied in this early stage of Sclerosis, our remedy will enable the maturer stages to be avoided. It proves effective, however, in the later stages too. (Detailed instructions are included with the preparation.)

2. " *Bidor* " *as a Remedy for Migraine*

The head-system is so constituted that the internal greyish-white portion of the brain (the " white matter ") represents physically the most highly advanced member of the human organization. This portion of the brain contains the sensory activity, in which the remaining activities of the senses are gathered up, and into which the Ego and astral body pour their forces. It shares also in the rhythmic system of the body, into which the astral body and the etheric are working. Lastly, it partakes, though to a very small extent, in the metabolic and limbs system in which the physical and etheric body make their influences felt. This part of the brain is different from the surrounding periphery (the " grey matter "), which contains in its physical constitution far more of the metabolic and limbs system, somewhat more of the rhythmic system, and least of all of the nerves-and-senses system. Now if, owing to a repressed activity of the Ego-organization, the nervous and sensory activity in the interior of the brain is impoverished and the digestive enhanced —*i.e.*, if the interior becomes more like the periphery of the brain than in the normal state— Migraine arises. The cure of this ailment will, therefore, depend: 1. On a stimulation of the activity of the nerves and senses; 2. On the transformation of a rhythmic activity that inclines to the metabolism into one that inclines more to the breathing process; and 3. On a restraint of the purely vegetative metabolic activity which is unregulated by the organization of the Ego. The first of these results is attained by the use of silica. Silicon, in combination with oxygen, contains processes equivalent to those that take place, within the organism, in the transition from the breathing to the activity of nerves and senses. The second result is to be achieved through sulphur, which contains processes whereby the rhythm that inclines to the digestive system is transformed into a rhythm that inclines to the breathing. Lastly, the third effect is attained by the use of iron, which conveys the metabolism immediately afterwards into the rhythmic process of the blood, whereby the metabolic process as such is restrained. Iron, sulphur, and silica, properly combined and administered, must therefore represent a remedy for Migraine. We have found this confirmed in countless cases.

3. A Remedy for Tracheitis and Bronchitis—Iron Pyrites

The medicament we will now discuss owes its existence to the perception which is able rightly to relate the processes, inherent in the substances of Nature, to those in the human organism. In this connection we must bear in mind that a substance is really a process brought to a standstill, a frozen process, as it were. Properly speaking we should say, not " pyrites," but " pyrites-process." The process which is thus fastened or frozen, as it were, in the mineral pyrites, represents what can result from the co-operation of the several processes of iron and sulphur. Iron, as we saw in the previous section, stimulates the circulation of the blood, while sulphur mediates for the connection of the circulation and the breathing. Now the origin of tracheitis and bronchitis, and of certain kinds of impediment of speech, lies at the very point where the circulation and the breathing come into mutual relation. This process between the circulation and the breathing (it is the process whereby the corresponding organs are created in the embryo period, and re-created again and again in the further course of life) can be taken over, if it is not working normally, by the iron-sulphur substance introduced into the body from outside. Starting from this perception, we prepare a remedy for the above forms of disease out of the mineral pyrites. In preparation of the remedy, the mineral is so transformed that its forces can find their way (internal treatment being indicated) into the diseased organs. We must, of course, have knowledge of the paths which certain substance-processes will take within the body. The metabolism carries the iron-process into the circulation of the blood; the sulphur-process passes on from the circulation into the breathing.

4. *Effects of Antimony Compounds*

Antimony has an extraordinarily strong affinity to other bodies, such, for instance, as sulphur. It thus reveals that it will readily accompany sulphur on the path which the latter takes through the organism—into all the breathing processes, for example. A further property of antimony is its tendency to radiant or starry forms of crystallization. Here it shows how easily it follows certain radiations of forces in the Earth's environment. This property becomes more evident when antimony is subjected to the Seiger process, whereby it assumes a fine and delicate texture. Still more significantly, it appears when antimony is brought into the process of combustion. The white smoke which it evolves, deposited on cold surfaces, forms the very characteristic " flowers of antimony." Now just as antimony gives itself up to the forces that work upon it when it is outside the human organism, so too, it follows the form-giving forces when it is within. In the blood, there is, as it were, a state of equilibrium between the form-giving and form-dissolving forces. By virtue of its properties above described, antimony can carry the form-creating forces of the human organism into the blood, if the way is prepared for it by combination with sulphur. The forces of antimony are indeed the very forces that work in the coagulation of the blood. To spiritual science the process appears as follows: The astral body is strengthened in the forces leading to the coagulation of the blood. For we must recognize in the antimony-forces and in the astral body similar forces which work in the organism centrifugally,

163

from within outward. These antimonizing forces oppose the forces, directed from without inward, which liquefy the blood and place the liquefied blood plastically in the service of the formation of the body. In the direction of these latter forces, those of albumen are also working. The forces contained in the albuminous process do in fact perpetually hinder the coagulation of the blood. Take the case of typhoid fever. It is due to a preponderating influence of the albuminizing forces. If antimony is administered in very minute doses, the forces that give rise to typhoid fever are counteracted. It must, however, be borne in mind that the effect of antimony is altogether different according as it is applied internally or externally. Applied externally, in ointments and the like, it weakens those centrifugal forces of the astral body which express themselves for instance in the symptoms of eczema. Internally administered it counteracts the excessive centripetal forces which manifest themselves in typhoid fever, for example.

Antimony is an important remedy in all diseases accompanied by a dangerous lowering of consciousness or somnolence. Here the formative centrifugal forces of the astral body, and hence also the processes of the brain and the senses, are to some extent out of action. If antimony is administered,

164

the deficient astral forces are artificially engendered. We shall always observe that the absorption of antimony strengthens the memory, enhances the creative powers, and generally improves the inner poise and composure of the soul. From the strengthened soul the organism is regenerated. In the older medicine this was felt to be so, and antimony was thus regarded as a universal medicament. And if this extreme standpoint is no longer ours, nevertheless, as will be seen from the above, we cannot but perceive in antimony a many-sided remedy.

5. *Cinnabar*

We have found cinnabar a valuable remedy. This substance affords a good opportunity of studying the relationship, so frequently alleged and no less frequently disputed, of mercury to the organization of man. Mercury is once more a " frozen process "; it stands in the very midst of the reproductive processes which, working within the organism, detach themselves almost entirely from its existence.

The mercury forces have the peculiar property of bringing about a re-absorption of these detached forces into the organism as a whole. Therapeutically mercury may therefore be applied (in very minute doses, needless to say) when there are processes arising in the organism which tend to become detached and separated out of the organism as a whole, and need to be brought back under its dominion. All catarrhal processes are of this kind. They arise when, by some external agency, one or other tract within the body is torn away from the dominion of the whole. This is the case, for example, with tracheitis and other catarrhal symptoms in the same region. Mercury forces, conveyed to this part of the body, will have a curative effect. We have referred already to the characteristic property of sulphur, which makes its influence felt in that domain of the organism where the circulation and the breathing processes meet— that is to say, in all that proceeds from the lungs. Cinnabar, as a compound of mercury and sulphur, is therefore an effective remedy for all catarrhal symptoms in these regions.

6. "*Gencydo*" *as a Remedy for Hay Fever*

The morbid symptoms of Hay Fever represent an inflammatory condition of the mucous membranes of the eyes, the nose, the throat, and upper air-passages. The past history of the patient generally indicates that he suffered already in childhood from diseased processes which may be included in the term "exudative diathesis." These indications point to the etheric body and to the abnormal behaviour of the astral. The etheric body is preponderating in its forces, while the astral body withdraws and shows a disinclination to take proper hold of the etheric and physical. The catarrhal symptoms result from the fact that in the parts diseased the regular influence of the astral body, and hence, too, of the Ego-organization, is disturbed. The astral body and Ego-organization become hypersensitive, which explains the sudden attacks and spasmodic reactions to sense-impressions: to light, to heat and cold, to dust, etc.

A healing process for Hay Fever must therefore come to the assistance of the astral body, helping it to enter in and take proper hold of the etheric. This can be done by the aid of the juices of fruits that possess a leathery skin or rind. We need only look at these fruits in a true way, to realize how strongly they are subject to form-creating forces of the kind that work from without inwards. Applying the juices of such fruits externally and internally, we can stimulate the astral body and urge it in the direction of the etheric. In the mineral constituents of the fruit-juices (potassium, calcium, and silica, for example) this influence receives further support from the side of the Ego-organization (*cf.* Chap. XVII). In this way a real cure of hay fever is effected. (Detailed instructions are included with the preparation.)

AFTERWORD

THUS far the fruits of our common work; and at this point, to the great grief of us all, the writing had to be discontinued when Rudolf Steiner's illness began. In the sequel it had been our plan to describe what works, by way of earthly and cosmic forces, in the metals gold, silver, lead, iron, copper, mercury, and tin, and to explain how these are to be applied in the art of healing. It was also our intention to describe how the ancient Mysteries contained a deep and true understanding of the relation of the metals to the planets, and their relations again to the various organs of the human body. To speak of this kind of Knowledge, to lay the foundations of it once more for our own time—such was our purpose.

It will be my task in the near future, from the notes and verbal indications that were given me, to compile and publish the second volume.—I.W.

NOTE

FOR the convenience of the medical profession and others interested in the development of Anthroposophical Therapy, arrangements have been made for the distribution of the medicaments prepared by the Clinical and Therapeutic Institute, and the " ILAG " Laboratories of Arlesheim-Dornach, Switzerland, through a London agency

THE BRITISH WELEDA CO. LTD.,

    21 Bloomsbury Square, London, W.C.1,

where full particulars can be obtained on application.